CRITICAL QUALITATIVE HEALTH RESEARCH

Critical Qualitative Health Research seeks to deepen understandings of the philosophies, politics and practices shaping contemporary qualitative health-related research. This accessible, lively, controversial introduction draws on current empirical examples and critical discussion to show how qualitative research undertaken in neoliberal healthcare contexts emerges and the range of complex issues qualitative researchers confront.

This book provides readers with an interrogative discussion of the histories and the legacies of qualitative research as well as the more recent calls for renewed criticality and demands for activism in research to respond to global health concerns. Contributions further showcase a range of contemporary work engaging with these issues and the encounters with philosophies, politics and practices this involves; from seeking explicit engagements with more recent posthuman ideas, as well as detailed and revised explorations of deeply engaged humanist approaches, to further critical discussions of the politics and practices of novel, digital and creative methods.

This book offers postgraduate researchers, health researchers and students opportunities to engage with the emergent and messy terrain of qualitative health-related research.

Kay Aranda is a Reader in the School of Health Sciences at the University of Brighton. Having worked in primary care, public health and community health nursing, her research interests include theory-informed qualitative and feminist research and inequalities related to gender, age and sexuality.

The introduction to this text promises a different perspective on qualitative research in healthcare, and its readers will not be disappointed. It takes a critical stance, and a discussion of the philosophical and political dimensions illuminates the complexities of this type of inquiry which is sometimes forgotten in other texts. The authors are known scholars and researchers in the field of health and social sciences research with a wide range of publications between them.

Immy Holloway, Professor Emeritus, Faculty of Health and Social Sciences, Bournemouth University, UK

This edited volume maps contrasting routes to doing empirical qualitative research in health and social care contexts. It critically examines how knowledge is always contested, partial, perspectival and imbued with power relations. Kay Aranda, and her impressive gathering of diverse researcher-practitioners, do a fine job in responding to the call for researchers to be more explicitly reflexive about their choices. Authors explain their preferred methodological and epistemological paths and argue their vision of a society that prioritises anti-oppressive civic values over divisive positivist and market-led ideology. This is a timely contribution, reminding us all to care, question our philosophical assumptions, and engage in critical political debate. This philosophically-informed volume will be an invaluable resource for any doctoral student seeking direction through the bewildering terrain of contemporary qualitative methodologies.

Dr Linda Finlay, PhD, BA(Hons)Psych, MBPsS,DipIntPsych, DipPCSup, Integrative Psychotherapist and Academic Consultant

This is a very interesting and impressive book focusing on critical qualitative research in healthcare, acknowledging the problematic of power and inequalities in how qualitative research has been and is designed from the perspective of the researcher as well as the research participants and the topics and issues researched. There is a great deal in this book for those engaged in qualitative research. The book supports new and novel approaches to qualitative research and this is a refreshing aspect for those looking for new ways to undertake qualitative research. In particular, I liked the consistent theme of co- producing research including the engagement and involvement of lay people and services users at all stages of the research. This is an important book for those who are using or plan to use qualitative research methodologies and it provides many examples of how to carry out credible and rigorous qualitative research.

Dr Anne Arber, Senior Lecturer, School of Health Sciences, University of Surrey, Guildford, UK

CRITICAL QUALITATIVE HEALTH RESEARCH

Exploring Philosophies, Politics and Practices

Edited by Kay Aranda

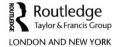

LONDON AND NEW YORK

First published 2020
by Routledge
2 Park Square, Milton Park, Abingdon, Oxon OX14 4RN

and by Routledge
52 Vanderbilt Avenue, New York, NY 10017

Routledge is an imprint of the Taylor & Francis Group, an informa business

© 2020 selection and editorial matter, Kay Aranda; individual chapters, the
contributors

The right of Kay Aranda to be identified as the author of the editorial material,
and of the authors for their individual chapters, has been asserted in accordance
with sections 77 and 78 of the Copyright, Designs and Patents Act 1988.

All rights reserved. No part of this book may be reprinted or reproduced or
utilised in any form or by any electronic, mechanical, or other means, now
known or hereafter invented, including photocopying and recording, or in any
information storage or retrieval system, without permission in writing from the
publishers.

Trademark notice: Product or corporate names may be trademarks or registered
trademarks, and are used only for identification and explanation without intent to
infringe.

British Library Cataloguing in Publication Data
A catalogue record for this book is available from the British Library

Library of Congress Cataloging-in-Publication Data
A catalog record has been requested for this book

ISBN: 978-1-138-36122-5 (hbk)
ISBN: 978-1-138-36126-3 (pbk)
ISBN: 978-0-429-43277-4 (ebk)

Typeset in Bembo
by Taylor & Francis Books

CONTENTS

List of figures	*vii*
List of tables	*viii*
List of boxes	*ix*
List of contributors	*xi*
Preface	*xiv*

Introduction	1
Kay Aranda	
1 Qualitative research and ideological pragmatism?	25
Chris Cocking	
2 Case study methodology	41
Kay de Vries	
3 Qualitative methods: Challenges and celebrations of fieldwork in the health care setting	53
Julie Scholes	
4 The practice of grounded theory: An interpretivist perspective	71
Julie Scholes	
5 Engaging with grounded theory research as a doctoral student	91
Heather Baid	
6 From phenomenology to practice: Theoretical foundations and phenomenological methods	110
Kate Galvin, Oliver Thurlow and Rebecca Player	

vi Contents

7 Phenomenology – questioning consciousness and experience   125
   Graham Stew

8 Rethinking ethnography with practice theory: Engaging with
   critical theory in qualitative health research   142
   Debbie Hatfield

9 Autoethnography   159
   Alec Grant

10 Postcritical qualitative feminist research: Implications for
    participatory and narrative approaches   177
    Kay Aranda

11 The reflexive autoethnographer   196
    Alec Grant

Index   *214*

FIGURE

5.1 Initiating the research process from a philosophical
positioning 92

TABLES

4.1	Analytical variance	77
5.1	Activities to develop ontological and epistemological positioning	93
5.2	Grounded theory terminology	95
5.3	Dimensional analysis table template	96
5.4	Dimension table example	97
5.5	Dimensional analysis summary table example	99
5.6	Microsoft Office Word skills to help postgraduate students	106

BOXES

0.1	Multiple social worlds: multiple ontological properties	6
2.1	Examples of cases in research on dementia	42
2.2	Ethnographic approach	43
2.3	Example of propositions for a study on dementia care in hospital	44
2.4	Examples of case boundaries	46
2.5	Triangulation exemplars	47
2.6	Example of presentation of multiple cases and cross-case analysis	50
3.1	Pragmatic checklist when deciding the interview location	56
3.2	Email interviews	59
3.3	Example: tales from the field	63
3.4	Example: The simulation laboratory as proxy for the natural setting	65
3.5	Example: the practice of collaboration – finding a place for qualitative methods to empower the voice of people for whom the research is both for and about	67
4.1	Example: objectivism – constructivism	75
4.2	Reflexive interrogation	83
4.3	Organising data	84
4.4	When to review the literature	85
	Editing	86
	Impact	87
8.1	Characteristics of focused ethnography	152
9.1	My brother was very fat	161

x List of boxes

9.2	Othering	162
9.3	Whose story is it?	163
9.4	Narrative entrapment	166
9.5	Conventional qualitative inquiry	167
9.6	Narrative recovery	168
9.7	Drinking to relax	170
9.8	Function or flavor?	171
9.9	Moral evaluation	172
11.1	The reflexivity koan	197
11.2	Drinking to relax	200
11.3	Ethical concerns	200
11.4	New materialist analysis	201
11.5	Demonstrating strong reflexivity	202
11.6	Demonstrating intersectional reflexivity	204
11.7	Demonstrating diffraction and narrative reflexivity	207
11.8	Toilets are the proper place for outputs	210

CONTRIBUTORS

Dr Kay Aranda is a Reader in the School of Health Sciences. Having studied social sciences, she then worked in community health nursing, health promotion and public health and in primary care and the voluntary sector in women's health. She has been an academic researcher for nearly 20 years, supporting postgraduate students in studying qualitative research, community health nursing and health inequalities, especially related to intersectional differences (e.g. gender, age, sexuality). She has more recently been involved in exploring feminist new materialisms, sociomaterial practice theories together with civil society community organisations. She has published widely on community nursing, resilience in relation to health inequalities and community health, as well as in relation to gender and sexuality and the use of feminist theories and concepts in healthcare for qualitative researchers.

Dr Heather Baid is a senior lecturer in critical care in the School of Health Sciences, University of Brighton. Currently, she leads the Intensive Care Pathway and BSc (Hons) Acute Clinical Practice degree for post-registration health care professionals. Her teaching regularly draws from qualitative research, and she also supports dissertation students to learn about qualitative methodology and methods. Heather has experience conducting qualitative research from her successfully completed PhD research project which was a constructivist grounded theory study about sustainability in critical care practice. She co-leads a specialist interest group on grounded theory in the School which provides a programme of seminars, support and expertise to early career and postgraduate researchers.

Dr Chris Cocking's research background is in the field of Social Psychology and involves the study of collectives and groups, falling into two main areas: crowd behaviour and collective resilience. His main body of interest is explaining how xii List of contributors

people behave in crowds and is part of a group of Social Psychologists who seem to spend a lot of their time overcoming the classic myths associated with collectives, as crowds often behave much better than they are usually given credit for. His own specific area of interest is mass emergency behaviour and how this influences disaster planning and response guidelines. What is increasingly emerging is that communities affected by emergencies are often much more resilient to adversity than was previously expected, and this has profound implications for emergency policy and planning. More recently, Chris has been looking at how people can come together if they have a shared experience of adversity, and how this collective resilience might also help mitigate the effects of exposure to stress. He has explored the emergence of collective resilience in a variety of diverse groups, such as nurses, paramedics, and young people at school dealing with the everyday stresses of growing up.

Kay de Vries is Professor of Older People's Health at De Montfort University, UK. She has a background in nursing and her early clinical practice was primarily in the community and hospice. Kay is predominantly a qualitative researcher and has expertise in all qualitative research methodologies and is also experienced in using mixed methods approaches. She has used Case Study methodology for many years and supervised several PhD students using this methodology. Kay has developed and led a number of postgraduate research programmes and supervised a large number of MSc and PhD research students to completion. Her research has predominantly focused on people with dementia and their family members; in acute, community and care home environments, and at end of life.

Oliver Thurlow and **Rebecca Player** are both postgraduate researchers undertaking doctoral funded fellowships in the School of Health Sciences at the University of Brighton, exploring health and well-being through lifeworld perspectives and descriptive phenomenology.

Professor Kathleen Galvin has been undertaking qualitative research for over 20 years and has been developing phenomenological oriented theoretical work in addition to empirical studies using phenomenology in a range of health and social care issues. This includes contributions to new perspectives of well-being, its absence and human dignity. She has been supervising candidates undertaking research degrees since 1997 and is still learning about the developing edge of phenomenological research and its potential.

Alec Grant, PhD is now an independent scholar, having retired from his position as Reader in Narrative Mental Health in the School of Health Sciences at the University of Brighton in May 2017. He is widely published in the fields of ethnography, autoethnography, and narrative inquiry. He was for some years the leader of the University of Brighton's postgraduate module, NAM13 *Qualitative Research,* and has taught autoethnography on that module for many years.

Dr Debbie Hatfield is a nurse and qualified teacher and has worked in healthcare education for over 25 years. She was a senior lecturer at the School of Health Sciences, University of Brighton for 20 years teaching on undergraduate and postgraduate pre- and post-registration courses. Initially working in critical and acute care, her interests later shifted to public health, service user involvement and community engagement. She has published and presented on clinical skills assessment, humanising healthcare and volunteering as part of the social engagement agenda within universities. In January 2014, Debbie secured a PhD studentship at Brighton and Sussex Medical School sponsored by the Higher Education Academy. Her research explored partnership working between service users and clinicians to commission and lead health and care services. Particularly the features of effective models of service user–clinician engagement and how this can impact the design of health care curricula. She has since successfully completed her PhD which was supervised by Professor Gordon Ferns, Dr Kay Aranda and Breda Flaherty.

Dr Julie Scholes (Consultant and Independent Researcher). Julie has been practising research, in particular grounded theory, since 1987 and teaching research methodology, philosophy and method since 1993. She has extensive experience of undertaking commissioned health care research in a variety of settings ranging from the critical care environment to mental health and community locations as well as educational settings. She has been supervising research degree students since 1995 and is constantly learning from her students how to address the challenges inherent in fieldwork, analysis and writing. Her research interests include how practitioners acquire expertise, aspire to caring excellence, and learn the art of nursing working with the participants of the research. She has a particular interest in involving patients and the public in research that is authentic and realistic and recently has been working with colleagues in the field of regenerative medicine. Now she is working at the Royal Hospital for Neurodisability working with colleagues to undertake research that focuses on the experience of patients and their families who experience complex and enduring long-term neurological disabilities.

Dr Graham Stew has worked in Higher Education for the last 30 years, and has a background in mental health and general nursing. Recently retired from his principal lecturer post in the School of Health Sciences at the University of Brighton, he is now an Associate Lecturer for the Open University. His research interests include inter-professional education, change management, reflective practice and mindfulness teaching. He currently supervises doctoral students and teaches research methodologies to postgraduate Open University students. Graham has a personal interest in non-dual teachings and has published four books on the subject. His main research expertise lies in the field of phenomenology, hermeneutics, interpretative phenomenological analysis and the philosophy of qualitative research.

PREFACE

The aim of this book is to explore the many ways in which philosophies, politics and practices enter into and shape the endeavour of qualitative research conducted in health-related settings. This edited collection is distinctive in aiming to engage with these facets of qualitative research at a time when questions over the value of qualitative research are evident, but yet when so many pressing global healthcare concerns over undignified or damaging care, growing inequalities and suffering, mental health issues, and increasing exclusions and marginalisation of minority communities and vulnerable of peoples, requires detailed, rich and in-depth accounts as well as challenging and troubling approaches. This book is further unique in offering contributions from a range of qualitative researchers confronting these issues, from early career to established experienced researchers and authors. The book aims to offer a critical counterpoint to current times. It provides an accessible, lively and controversial introduction to the diverse philosophies, politics and practices informing qualitative health-related research, aiming to open up these concerns for scrutiny/interrogation and to stimulate further inquiry and debate.

INTRODUCTION

Kay Aranda

The current contexts in which health, care and illness are researched have never been more troubling. A decade of global austerity measures, further intensified by neoliberal imperatives in healthcare, has led to an unprecedented rise in inequality, precarity and suffering (Dorling, 2015; Piketty, 2014). These contexts and concerns are well known to those working and researching in healthcare in the global north. This manifests in healthcare for example, as lives lost to poverty, disadvantage, exclusion, marginalisation, or is evident in daily experiences of suffering or harm from undignified, disrespectful and damaging treatment or care. Moreover, efforts to stay well or healthy or enhance mental and physical wellbeing are increasingly difficult to achieve in contexts and environments that are non-conducive and damaging people's health. With the rise of populist politics challenging democratic values of inclusion, equality and community solidarity, fears over widening social divisions and growing intolerance increase, issues which have in turn led to serious questions over the direction, purpose and value of public research (Buroway, 2015; Lather & St Pierre, 2013). One outcome has been to demand qualitative researchers take up more explicitly political positions, both in order to give attention to diverse experiences of vulnerability, precarity and disadvantage or health and wellbeing, but also to develop and defend a particular future vision of society that values and prioritises civic society over market or state (Buroway, 2015). This call demands increased activism that makes a tangible difference in people's lives, addressing suffering and social injustices in more relevant, detailed and convincing ways (Denzin, 2017; Flick, 2017; Lather, 2016). These contexts and uncertain times also mean that what is considered to be true or trustworthy, or what counts as credible knowledge, used to justify action or demands for change, remains deeply contested. Therefore, to seek to argue for deepening and developing our understandings of qualitative research in such contexts is both timely and political.

This edited collection aims to provide readers with a critical counterpoint to current times. Rather than endorsing naive or an uncritical engagement with qualitative research in healthcare settings, this collection shows instead the myriad ways in which researchers constantly search, adapt, improvise, extend, question, challenge, undo and revise normative thinking and practices governing qualitative research. This accessible, lively and controversial introduction to many of the diverse philosophies, politics and practices informing qualitative research reveals the continuing contested nature of knowledge, the constantly evolving politics and new forms of power relations involved in these endeavours. To question who research is for, and why, and how it takes place, or whose voices are made visible, ignored or heard, are part of the everyday practices of qualitative researchers and this book opens up these concerns for scrutiny and interrogation to stimulate further inquiry and debate.

Critique enables an opening up of phenomena in order to question the taken for granted, reveal hidden assumptions, and the operation of taken for granted or normative ideologies or discourses at work in everyday interactions, practice and/or relationships; it allows us to not only question, but ask further often difficult questions, or helps us rethink or reimagine what qualitative health research is, can, or should become. The following chapters and contributions showcase a range of qualitative researchers confronting these issues, from early career to developing and well-established experienced researchers and authors. All are healthcare academics/practitioners who are more than familiar with the worlds of healthcare that many postgraduate and researching practitioners face day-to-day.

This is a text specifically written for those postgraduate students and researchers in these challenging settings. It aims to address a distinct set of needs, voiced by increasing numbers of students, who express a desire to expand their understandings and knowledge beyond Western notions of positivistic approaches or mixed methodologies currently endorsed in national governments research programmes, which guide the direction and set priorities for funding and subsequent healthcare related research. From our experiences and our work with many postgraduate health research students, there is a wish instead to explore qualitative research both at introductory levels, as well as engage with the philosophical or theoretical complexities and politics informing methodologies, methods or practices of such. Though often intertwined and embedded in many discussions of methodologies and methods, these aspects of qualitative health research can be overlooked in a necessary desire to first learn more about the basic processes or techniques. Though primarily for postgraduate researchers and students, we hope this book is also of interest to undergraduate students or those with first degrees who wish to and are prepared to read 'beyond' introductory texts.

Themes

This introductory chapter explains why an approach to critical qualitative research in healthcare, exploring philosophies, politics and practices, is necessary. We start from a shared premise that, though passionate about these approaches, in all variations, qualitative research is not a given good. Qualitative research retains troubling past histories and legacies that still shape debates over its role and value and our choices over underlying philosophies, politics and practices today. In this introduction I aim to provide a brief overview of these complex critical histories of qualitative research in order to highlight a number of themes found throughout the contributions. I first discuss the nature and rationales for qualitative research in researching health related concerns and then review critical histories of qualitative research before moving on to consider more specifically the nature of philosophies, politics and practices in such work. In debating critical qualitative research, Flick (2017, p. 4), helpfully outlines a number of key ways in which criticality enters qualitative research and these are evident in the contributions to this book, with the third means often being the most challenging to achieve:

1. Inquiry can be critical about the issues that are studied – starting from a social, political or other problem, which should be addressed, and research should provide a critical perspective about.
2. We can be critical about the methods and approaches we use in our research – critical about other forms (like quantitative research) or about the established mainstream of qualitative research (or some parts of it).
3. A major challenge, however, is how to remain able in the light of the first two challenges to really do empirical qualitative research contributing to addressing social problems and to remain reflexive about what we do.

Qualitative research in healthcare or qualitative health research

In exploring qualitative research and healthcare, it is worth noting the debates over whether researchers merely use qualitative research as derived from social sciences, and transfer or apply to different settings, or whether qualitative research in these settings is different or distinctive. Qualitative health research is argued by some to be a distinctive subdiscipline of qualitative research (Morse, 2012), because of its specific aims to explore health and illness from the perspective of people, rather than from the clinicians' or researchers' viewpoints. Indeed Morse (2012), further suggests qualitative health research is uniquely defined by this focus on a health–illness continuum, using methods that are mainly inductive. Other scholars think of qualitative research as specific but suitably applied in healthcare settings (Holloway & Galvin, 2017) or argue for the range of specific qualitative methods used in health research (Green & Thorogood, 2018). This collection spans the range of these definitions.

Qualitative research in healthcare settings is arguably applied in one of two main ways. First, are the more familiar studies informing health and illness understandings, beliefs and the labour or work involved, providing the knowledge or evidence base upon which much health and illness knowledge, practice or treatment is based. Second, are the critical studies of health and illness, often more sociologically informed, that question the very concepts or explanations that constitute understandings of health or illness at any given time and place (Green & Thorogood, 2018). In sum, qualitative research related to healthcare or qualitative health research is broadly defined as forms of inquiry concerning the organisations, patterns, processes, including experiences and meanings of care and treatment, and the relations involved in understanding health and illness in a society. Qualitative health research draws on the specific strengths and distinctive nature of qualitative research to more specifically explore and account for understandings, beliefs, practices and experiences of health and/or illness, as well as the experiences and organisations of health services or care. It is also argued to include the histories, policies, workforce structure and design, as well as the type of knowledge generated and utilised by medicine, nursing, midwifery and allied health professions (Green & Thorogood, 2018). For the purposes of this collection the terms qualitative and qualitative health research will be used interchangeably.

Rationales for qualitative health research include attention to others' experiences, their involvement and engagement in the process to gather and generate a shared account of histories or needs. With its ability to capture the specific and particular rather than the general or universal, qualitative research is arguably especially suited to healthcare research because of its ability to explore the unique, rich, in-depth meanings and details of people's lives (Taylor & Francis, 2013). Thus one of the strengths is to offer in-depth, detailed explorations of people's complex subjective experiences of health, illness or disabling or chronic conditions, offering detailed insights and knowledge with which to design or deliver more affirming, appropriate and responsive care (Holloway & Galvin, 2017; Galvin & Todres, 2011). Indeed, many argue that qualitative health research offers specific methods necessary to the contexts of health, care and illness, and emphasise the range of methodologies that are particularly well suited to practitioner researchers' worlds of healthcare research, where communication, interaction and caring may be prioritised. Qualitative research can therefore be said to offer new ways to explore and understand the complex worlds of health and illness (Bourgeault, Dingwell, & De Vries, 2010; Pope & Mays, 2006).

Most definitions of qualitative research emphasise how inquiry seeks to generate knowledge about meanings, feelings, behaviours, perceptions people ascribe to their lives and experiences (Leavy, 2017). Drawing on these subjective accounts, qualitative researchers develop in-depth understandings, immersing themselves in the natural settings of people's worlds and lives; they aim to focus on emic perspectives or the insider view of people, their perceptions, meanings, interpretations and understandings by generating rich, detailed complex data. Working inductively, to generate such meaning and detail means qualitative designs are malleable and revisable as learning develops and the research unfolds (Hesse-Biber & Leavy, 2008; Leavy, 2017). As such, these detailed descriptions of phenomena claim to be grounded in participants perspectives (Ritchie, Lewis, McNaughton Nicholls, & Ormston, 2014). Analysis of these accounts seek to retain complexity and nuance, often working with iterative interpretation that aims to remain open to emergent categories and themes, aiding the development of theories, strategies and actions. The focus is on holistic approaches which are methodological and theoretically diverse and where choices of methods or methodology are informed by philosophies that provide a framing, or paradigm and worldview that guides the research project (Leavy 2017). Systematically and rigorously conducted, yet flexible and contextual, qualitative research is therefore argued to be capable of producing explanations and arguments. Finally, practices of reflexivity, transparency and criticality aim to ensure qualitative research is accountable in being able to resonate, be credible and recognisable to those whose lives are involved and through self-scrutiny and questioning of the whole research endeavour, its quality and aims, and thus remains a moral and political practice.

Why use qualitative research in healthcare research?

Qualitative research is considered particularly pertinent to health research at present for several reasons. First, qualitative ways of researching have a unique but critical contribution to make to questions of experience, challenging whose knowledge matters. The growing agenda of service user involvement in health, though not without its own political and moral challenges (Wilson et al., 2015), is nevertheless changing dominant paradigms of research previously driven by professionals' interests and concerns (Locock, Boylan, Snow, & Staniszewska, 2017; Boote & Booth, 2015). This engagement and involvement of the public and patients attempts to alter the balance of power over what constitutes knowledge and expertise (Beresford, 2013). This agenda is well suited to qualitative research and recent reviews have found this to be so (Boote & Booth, 2015). Insisting on the value and importance of experience and participation from the perspective of those communities affected and/or the grassroots and social movements that have sought redress or provide alternative provision, has meant involvement, engagement and participation have become central to policy and research practice in the UK in the NHS, and globally (Slutsky et al., 2016; National Standards for Public Involvement in Research 2018).

Secondly, there is recognition that healthcare practitioners' encounters with individuals, families or communities are founded upon generating life histories, stories and ongoing narratives through assessments, planning and engagements or interactions involved in delivering and receiving ongoing care. The resultant rise in qualitative, narrative-based research in health and social care research is therefore clearly evident in recent years (Andrew, Squires, & Tambourkou 2008; Hurwitz, Greenhalgh, & Skultans, 2004; Holloway & Freshwater, 2007). Further impetus towards more narrative and participatory research practices comes from a growing political intent to give voice to those excluded or made invisible, be it through lack of access to care or services or treatment. The lived experiences of those 'othered' or made vulnerable in health and care systems, such as children, young people, people living with mental health or learning disabilities, autism, or dementia have consequently substantially increased in recent years.

6 Kay Aranda

Finally, many issues practitioners come to research arise out of their encounters with people and care services, of something being absent, missing, problematic, as well as from their own personal politics, passions and desires to address social injustice. These profound troubling discomforts can drive demands for critical reflexive understandings of the self and others, but also for consideration of wider sociopolitical perspectives on the contexts in which healthcare unfolds and for which qualitative research is especially suited (Finlay & Ballinger, 2006). Often focused on differing aspects of social worlds of healthcare, as Mason and Dale (2011) suggest, qualitative research can offer rich multiple perspectives for viewing and understanding the worlds of health and care, given that these worlds can be comprised of many differing ontological properties (see Box 0.1).

BOX 0.1 MULTIPLE SOCIAL WORLDS: MULTIPLE ONTOLOGICAL PROPERTIES

Stories or interpretations
Socio-architectural structures and systems
Individuals, feelings, emotions
Behaviours, actions and events
Environmental, non-human or sensory world
Relationalities, connections and situations
Multiple and non-cohering realities

(Adapted from Mason & Dale, 2011).

The more recent renewed demand for a new critical qualitative research, which I discuss next, has emerged from this landscape (Denzin, 2017; Denzin & Lincoln, 2018; Flick, 2017). This call builds upon a further role of qualitative research to unsettle, undo, or trouble common sense understandings or knowledges, but also the practices and assumptions to doing research (Turner, Short, Grant, & Adams, 2018; Denzin, 2017; Lather, 2016). This is critical qualitative research that not only describes what or where or how something is happening but is inquiry with an overt political intent and interest in change.

Critical histories of qualitative and health-related research

Critical theory–informed qualitative research is often argued to originate from the critical theory developed by the Frankfurt School (Seidman, 2011; Seidman & Alexander, 2001). It was initiated and developed by Horkeheimer and others (Seidman, 2011), partly in response to frustrations with the failures of Marxism, and the political contexts giving rise to European fascism, then later, known under the label of new critical theory across the social sciences. These are theories to be found in the work of Habermas and Honneth (Honneth, 2007; Meehan, 1995), and similar important inspired strands of this thinking are evident in the initial Marxist then socialist inspired feminist theories of second wave feminism (Butler & Scott, 1992). Again later, critical theory is evident in the poststructuralism of Foucault and together with work encompassing poststructural feminism, queer, disability and critical race theory and black, postcolonial researchers (Hall, Jagose, Bebell, & Potter, 2013; Jagose, 2009; Lewis & Mills, 2003; Hekman, 1996; Foucault, 1980).

From this rich legacy of scholarly work, the grounds or foundations of all inquiry, including qualitative research, were increasingly recognised as being far from neutral, benign or innocent; instead, knowledge was argued to always arise from sets of interests and particular positions. All knowledge was argued to be partisan, partial and imbued with power relations, manifest as interests derived from specific perspectives on the world, which were and are themselves products of power and of time and place (Hekman, 1996; Flax, 1990). Claims of objectivity, distance or detachment, or measures to remove bias were therefore argued to be just that: claims or statements that served to disguise the extent to which sets of interests and partiality were and are embedded in all knowledge production.

The view from somewhere

The partiality of knowledge is evident in the dominant canons of thought to which novice qualitative health researchers are introduced. These are more often than not derived from a classical white, Western, Anglo American, Eurocentric tradition, with philosophies, politics and practices predominately produced by white, privileged men and their perspectives or voices, most usually based in relatively rich, developed or global north countries such as the USA or Europe, and frequently assumed to be unproblematic when applied in qualitative health research, even when the focus is international or global health concerns (Green & Thorogood, 2018). An uncritical use of this canon reinforces sets of assumptions about what is valued and which notions of reality are prioritised and which practices are endorsed such as objectivity, neutrality, distance. Linguistic binaries structure thought such as those between individual and the social, or collective, subject and object, male or female, public or private and personal, agency and structure and/or rationality or reason rather than emotion. These binaries serve to obscure or disguise both the partiality and normative superiority of one term other the other, and so the inherent privileging of rational scientific knowledges through supposed claims of objectivity and neutrality. One result of these binaries and assumptions is that tacit, indigenous, experiential, affective, narrative and performative ways of knowing are devalued or dismissed as being too partial, too subjective or emotional and even irrelevant to the main business of bringing about change in healthcare.

Voice and experience

A further challenge to qualitative research more recently is the question of the assumed unproblematic notion of capturing and representing experiences, or of giving voice to those marginalized, invisible or oppressed. From a poststructural perspective, the notion of reflecting back an authentic experience assumes a subject who can express free will through intentions, as found in action, language, and in the public sphere (St Pierre, 2009). To refuse this assumption builds upon the critical use of voice already present in qualitative researchers' work. Here experience is always more than a reflection of the real, instead voice or experience in qualitative research is understood as comprised of complex patterns of power and desire that are involved in speaking of, for and about others (Jackson & Mazzei, 2009). Moreover, as Joan Scott (1992) previously argued, as the basis for authoritative knowledge, an appeal to experience is extremely limited. With experience always already interpretation and not the origin of knowledge or the authoritative evidence for what is known, she argues it is the concept of experience that needs explaining. For what counts as experience is far from self-evident, she argues. Experience is always, already culturally constituted, contested and therefore political. Responses to similar challenges over questions of representation and voice can be found for example in queer, feminist and autoethnographic research, in later more social-constructionist/constructivists accounts of phenomenology and grounded theory as well as critical ethnography, where there is a recognition of a plurality of voice and attention to power relations is given and involves questioning who can speak for whom (Aranda, 2018; Turner et al., 2018, Browne & Nash, 2010).

Decolonising research

Further critical qualitative research approaches are to be found from those scholars exposing the inherent racism in Western epistemologies and research, and who argue for a decolonising of methodologies to develop spaces for indigenous methodologies (Mohanty, 1988; Hill Collins, 2000; Kovach, 2009; Lorde, 2007; hooks, 1982). In this critical tradition Western research, as the product of European imperialism, racism, and colonisation, contains the worst excesses of Western scientific research, all conducted in the name of progress (Smith, 2012). For example, anthropology then ethnography, was in its early forms complicit with seeking to classify, collect and represent knowledge about indigenous people's lives back to the West, and then back to indigenous peoples themselves; people's lives were constructed as somehow exotic, unknown, or in need of taming or civilising (Smith, 2012). These offensive histories and legacies of pain, suffering and abuse show Western research is far from being a given good in the world. Rather, it again substantiates just how far all inquiry is infused with privilege and power and partial, vested interests which are too often disguised as universal truths or claims of progress. Research is therefore a significant site between Western interests and the ways of resisting and knowing by the 'Other' (Smith, 2012). Decolonising methodologies seeks to unmask and deconstruct Western ideals of philosophy and political theory, such as emancipation or empowerment, revealing these intentions as specific products of Western liberal democratic thinking and ideologies. Falcón (2016) for example, favours a transnational feminism which would aim to decolonise and create new structures, institutions and models and practices, whereby qualitative researchers from the global north recognise and draw more widely from the many epistemological tools derived from indigenous, women of colour, as well as African descendants social movements from Latin America.

A new critical qualitative health research

Recent renewed interest in critique within the social sciences and demands for a renewed critical qualitative research converges with these aforementioned critiques. Many of the current demands for research to change are equally related to the epistemic turns or shifts away from formal grand theories or narratives across the social sciences. Here dominant knowledges are contested by those misrecognised, excluded or marginalised, or by those wanting to radically question who is positioned at the centre and as marginal, or whose experiences count as knowledge, together with those scholars and activists advocating with communities, arguing for meaningful transformative, egalitarian and emancipatory changes and ways of knowing (Denzin, 2017; Lather, 2016; Browne & Nash, 2010; Mertens, 2007; Ahmed, 2006). As Denzin (2017) suggests, these histories and traditions of critical research encompass many of the following philosophies, politics and practices:

> These individuals use participatory, constructivist, critical, feminist, queer, and critical race theory, and cultural studies models of interpretation. They locate themselves on the epistemological borders between postpositivism and poststructuralism. They work at the centers and the margins of intersecting disciplines, from communications, to race, ethnic, religious and women's studies, from sociology, history, anthropology, literary criticism, political science, and economics, to social work, health care, and education. They use multiple research strategies, from case study, to ethnography, phenomenology, grounded theory, biographical, historical, participatory, and clinical inquiry. As writers and interpreters, these individuals wrestle with positivist, postpositivist, poststructural, and postmodern criteria for evaluating their written work.
>
> *(p. 10)*

As noted at the start of this introduction, both Flick (2017) and Denzin (2017) argue current neoliberal cultures, with rising levels of precarity, huge disparities in wealth, opportunities and increasingly unliveable lives require forms of inquiry that explicitly address inequities through unsettling what counts as research or evidence. The critical approaches are similar to previous inceptions of critical theory in not only wanting to understand the world, but to challenge and change it. This renewed interest and impetus arises from our contemporary times. The neoliberal worlds of growing inequality and injustices means seeking transformative forms of research to achieve social justice (Mertens, 2009; Denzin, 2017).

10 Kay Aranda

Many of the more recent critical approaches draw upon poststructural, post-colonial, postfoundational understandings of theory and research (Aranda, 2018). The overall arguments for a new critical qualitative research (Flick, 2017; Charmaz, 2017; Lather & St Pierre, 2013), is to revitalise and make visible the foundations of previous critical approaches working in similar traditions, from feminism, post-colonial, minority ethnic and peoples of colour, queer, LGBTQ and disability activists, so that politics and practices unite as action or activism, and qualitative research is driven not by researchers interests, but by those of the most vulnerable, exploited or oppressed. The philosophies, politics and practices of contemporary qualitative research in healthcare are therefore complex and need exploring further.

Philosophies, politics and practices

Most introductions to qualitative research do not necessarily highlight these three complex interrelated terms. In this book, these terms help reframe our discussions of qualitative research. While seemingly distinct areas, they are in fact difficult to view separately given the ways they intersect and interact throughout the whole endeavour of research which I explore in more detail next.

Philosophies

Philosophy, for example, is a notoriously difficult term to sum up; given its many meanings, arguments and contested areas of specialism and with disciplines ranging from epistemology, logic, ethics, aesthetics, metaphysics and politics. However, qua-litative researchers are familiar with the questions philosophers ask, as these episte-mological and ontological questions about how we know what we know, or questions over what it is to be in the world, and the nature of that reality, are often the first introduction to the contested nature of epistemology and ontology and its relationship to theory and methodology. Furthermore, it is important to note that contemporary present-day philosophers continue to seek to address current concerns and social problems. This involves questions concerning the values and practices of liberal democracy, or in understanding political resistance, or questions over abuses of power, or more inclusive notions of equality or freedom; and finally, how suffering, pain, loss of self, vulnerability and misrecognition can be more urgently and ade-quately addressed (Butler, Gambetti, & Sabsay, 2016; Ranciere, 2010; Englemann, 2009; Butler, 2004a; Rorty, 1999; Agamben, 1998).

In classical times, from Plato, Aristotle and Socrates, the knowledge generated through rational thought and argument was considered to provide certain knowl-edge, offering foundations and guides for how people should live or how society might be organised to pursue social goods such as justice or the good life. This is the metaphysical approach to philosophy, aiming to understand and explain everything (Benton & Craib, 2001). An alternative, more modest view of philo-sophy accepts the premise that more secure knowledge comes from our rationality and senses, from practical experience, observation and given the use of reason, from scientific experimentation. Though comprised of many complex positions, positivism and notions of empiricism is helped by this analytical or rational school of philosophy by exposing and critiquing common sense thinking, unexamined assumptions, prejudices and biases. This approach to experiential knowledge builds upon and accepts the value of people's implicit everyday reflecting or philosophising, a philosophical orientation to the world we all use to navigate life or important emotional events or transitions and our relationships (Benton & Craib, 2001).

In contrast, though again, not without encompassing many overlapping, complex positions, broadly speaking there is a view of philosophy that emphasises the social, cultural and historical conditions of thought and existence. This is evident in what is termed continental as opposed to the above more analytical view of philosophy (West, 2010). Continental philosophy is borne out of a series of critiques of Western and European Enlightenment thinking, with its championing of science and scientific rationality, and instead seeks to question the search for and possibility of certain, secure foundations to knowledge. It is this latter set of philosophical approaches that inform the development of critical theories and critical qualitative research. As we have seen, based on critical theory from Marxism, the Frankfurt school, Habermas, feminism, phenomenology and poststructuralism for example, what emerges in qualitative inquiry are critical participatory, narrative and critical ethnographies/autoethnographies, critical feminist and critical phenomenological or queer research as well as critical decolonising methodologies or postcolonial research and critical discourse analysis and more (West, 2010). Thus any search for certainty and grand explanations or narratives is driven by Enlightenment thinking, whereby reason would ensure the modern world would move ever closer to progress and emancipation from past superstitions and irrational beliefs. Qualitative research, though part of this belief in modernity and the modern progressive turn, seeking to document or explore and interpret, or give voice to those most invisible or disadvantaged, has not done so uncritically as we have discussed previously.

With modernity and its assumptions severely challenged from the early twentieth century onwards by postmodern thought or postmodernism, these challenges were premised upon claims of the subsequent decline of traditional values, institutions, the questioning of scientific progress and failings of science, the superiority of scientific knowledge was severely disputed. The challenges, from scholars, like philosophers such as Foucault or Butler, viewed the modern world as increasingly conflictual, subjugating, marginalising and exploitative, but also diverse and plural, full of resistance and challenge and potential change, being continually created or constructed or made through embodied practices, language, power and knowledge; this meant social life was best understood through these processes and relations (Nicholson, 1990). Given these epistemological and ontological assumptions, relativist or multiple notions of realities, beings, identities and understandings of the world came to the fore (Flax, 1990). As we will see later in the contributions for this book, these many positions and philosophies inform and underpin qualitative research in differing ways, with many theories used in qualitative research as more formal expressions of these ideas, that are both implicit and explicitly present and cited in research (Crotty, 2003).

12 Kay Aranda

Exploring humanism and posthumanism

One overall theme arising from the aforementioned review of critical histories of qualitative health research are the mainly Western philosophical notions of humanism and engagements with differently informed knowledges such as indigenous, non-secular, spiritual, or eco and transglobal notions of living well, as the more recent notions of the more-than-human world emphasised in notions of posthumanism (Braidotti, 2013). Notions of humanism and posthumanism depict an evolving set of ideas, assumptions, discourses or meanings that can be found in both more familiar interpretative/constructionist qualitative health research approaches, but equally in recent critical and post critical qualitative research. This major overarching theme of humanism and posthumanism, or a more-than-human stance provides a framing logic for the sequence of the chapters in this book.

European Enlightenment and Western Humanism

The historical period of European thought, known as the Enlightenment from the 1500s onwards, formed a highly influential foundational account of the Western modern world. Though never a uniform movement, its development was marked by attempts to discover or reveal universal principles that could uncover the truths about the world. This search for knowledge was to replicate the transcendental but detached God's eye view and was thus opposed to knowledge or perspectives informed by particular groups or persons. These allegiances to objectivity and knowledge as free of the influences of politics and values was translated into the scientific method.

Humanism is a further defining characteristic of this period in modern Western thought. Humanism is a philosophy and ethics that places the human subject at the centre of concern and value in understanding social life and change; it emphasises the value and agency of humans and is centred on their needs, interests and abilities or concerns. Only humans, originally just men, were capable of creating and controlling the universe through their capacities of reason; this universal power of self-reflexive reason was to provide certain foundations to knowledge and shaped European culture and knowledge as hegemonic, with humans becoming the unique source of meaning, value, truth and being (Braidotti, 2013). In this tradition, the human subject becomes an agent of their own subjectivity or sense of self, with such agency or free will, they can act independently on the world. These assumptions of reason or agency presuppose a common, universal nature or essence to humanity. Moreover, using reason, this autonomous human being has the potential to emancipate them self and others (Flax, 1992). Through the use of reason, as manifest in the scientific method, certain and reliable knowledge could be produced to enable this emancipation or freedom from past dogmas and mystical beliefs and ensure progressive change. The possibility of reason's purity was ensured by the assumed separation of the body or bodily concerns from the mind; undisturbed by experiences or bodily concerns, allowed the mind of reason or rational thought to act as the reliable source

Introduction   13

of universal truth. In summary, the key Enlightenment modernist humanist assumption is of the authorial subject who is:

- The source of all knowledge, meaning, value and truth
- Autonomous, has agency or free will, is independent
- Can create, emancipate and control through the use of knowledge based on the use of reason
- Reason or Mind are separate from the Body so thought is uncontaminated by emotions
- Subject is an agent of their own subjectivity and self
- Shared nature/essence/fixed and stable, is universal.
- Dualisms or binary thinking – mind/body, nature/culture, subject/object
- Progress and improvement are only possible from the use of reason
- Shapes European culture and knowledge to become hegemonic

(Adapted from Braidotti, 2013)

Posthumanism

In contrast, posthumanism and posthuman thought includes work that has for the last twenty years or more questioned the boundaries that define the human world. For some it is the apparent antihumanism of earlier poststructural theories which is similar to what scholars refer to as transhuman or the more-than-human world. Critics of humanism, such as Foucault (1974), for example, saw humanism as an abstract, universal grand narrative, depicting Western forms of reason and human nature as superior and universal that was then used to dominate others as uncivilised. Philosophically, some refer to posthumanism as expanding areas of moral concern and extending subjectivities to include more than just human concerns or needs; it expands the focus of inquiry to be more inclusive of the non-human but sentient beings and of the material world. Here the historical concepts of human nature or what is assumed to be fixed or belonging to humans are interrogated; this challenges conventional understandings of subjectivity, identity or concepts of experience, care or ethics as unproblematic or evidently transparent. For example, situated ethical practices, when conceived in the more-than-human world, involving human and non-human concerns requires different attunements, commitments and obligations; ethics and care become expansive and inclusive. In these understandings, concepts of care and ethics become relational forces, distributed across a multiplicity of agencies, relations (human and non-human) and materials, enmeshed in networks to support 'non-exploitative forms of togetherness, but which cannot be imagined once and for all' (Puig de la Bellacasa, 2017, p. 14).

Posthumanism therefore rejects the anthropocentrism of modern thought, questions the assumptions of human sovereignty or exceptionalism as seen in the uniqueness of human beings, with their assumed right to use materials, nature, objects as instruments or tools to control the world. Instead, much posthuman thought seeks to place humans back into a world as but one other species. With technological developments questioning what it means to be human and notions of humans as hybrids, with embodied experiences extended by attachments to digital technologies, such as mobile phones for example, this blurring and entanglement of boundaries between humans and matter or the material world, further implies a need to interrogate taken for granted concepts in health and illness research and how we generate knowledge. As this collection shows, for research, and qualitative research in particular, this has meant questioning again and revising concepts such as agency, experience or subjectivity, as well as those dominant binaries or catgorisations of health or illness, subject or object and nature or culture as separate, bounded, or distinct, rather than seeing them as relationally generated and entangled (Lather, 2016; Barad, 2007). This aim is to develop new understandings of the subject and other, agency, reason and consciousness, or identity, subjectivity and the body and for our purposes, of health, illness and care (Gherardi, 2017; Braidotti, 2013; Schatzki, 2001). Feminist Donna Haraway (2008), reminds us, though, of the incomplete business of modernity, with so much suffering, disadvantage and inequality for so many, human and non-human beings alike, she fears talk of a post-era – often implying as it does some more superior notion of progress or understanding of the world, will mean we neglect what still needs to be attended to. She wants to reject the term posthumanism and prefers the term 'companion species' as she argues we are and always will be born, grow and live with and die connected to other non-human beings or species.

For Schaticki (2001), two types of posthumanism are discernible; one is an approach that seeks to become more inclusive of the non-human world, together with the human world, as both worlds codetermine, direct and shape each other. This in turn challenges conventional understandings of the social – as in no longer being just about relations between humans. The other form of posthumanism is to understand the world in which humans are no longer the central focus, or decentred, but do not remove the significance of humans for understandings or analyses. For example, in posthuman practice theory, the focus of study becomes not humans per se, but the practices to which they are recruited, sustain and are located within; it is these practices that constitute the central phenomena to be studied in order to understand fuller more complete notions of experience, meaning, agency, or change and of course the more than human world. For Gherardi (2017), posthumanist thought is evident in the theoretical developments in sociology, with actor network theory of Latour (2007), or Science and Technology Studies (STS), disrupting the assumed binaries of subject/object, with the conventional understandings of an instrumental use of objects or technologies. Instead, the challenge is to view materials as co-implicated in shaping human identities and wider social worlds. Theoretically and ontologically, this assumes or emphasises a symmetry between human and non-human worlds, together with a relational epistemology that emphasises attachments or relations between more than just other subjects. These entanglements of subject and objects, or the more-than-human-world is viewed as constantly emerging or becoming, so here notions of performativity become key. This is the world understood through actions or sets of practices, as constellations or nexuses of practices, and with this comes an understanding of subjects, identities or gender, epistemology,

Introduction **15**

power and ontology as distributed and performative, ideas often most closely associated with Judith Butler (2004b) and Foucault (1980).

Politics

The politics of research is clearly inherent to all the aforementioned debates and developments given that politics is a term best understood as being concerned with power, and in modern world terms, power and people. Theories of power suggest two main schools; possessive and non possessive – one group has or possesses power (in terms of resources or social or cultural capital) over another or a group. Alternatively, power is viewed as discursive fields or forces, sets of knowledges and power or practices that circulate everywhere, belonging within all relations, institutions, structures and processes and is therefore more distributed or networked (Watson, 2017; Lukes, 2005). These notions of politics and power are both in relation to notions of more formal, organised, public arenas and contexts, present and historical, where, for example, research relations, processes and institutions or structures are conceived, devised, conducted, prioritised or valued; as well as the power or politics of private, intimate personal lives involved with others and selves, where emotions, decisions or actions, questions of our identity, sense of self or subjectivity, relations with others, and the moral actions or dilemmas occur. In research, these political issues and concerns are always present, ranging from questions of why conduct research, to whose knowledge counts or matters, to who gets to speak for whom (Denzin & Giardina, 2015). There are also myriad ways in which questions of power enter into research assumptions, questions, designs, methods of data collection or analysis and in the secrets and silences of research, questions of morality and authority, over presenting, exchanging and translating knowledge into benefits for communities and people, or academies and researchers (Ryan-Flood & Gill, 2010). Additionally, the politics of research is evident in the rise of participatory, involvement and engagement approaches of civic society, communities, the public and patients. These movements and developments to varying degrees challenge the aims, benefits and direction and control over the research process (Palmer et al., 2018). Moreover, as we will see later in this introduction, with critical research, the whole enterprise of Western research, its power base, its institutions and structures, and dominance and ability to distort accounts of people's lives and experiences, are excesses and abuses of power yet to be redressed (Smith, 2012).

In relation to qualitative research, politics is further seen, as we have discussed previously, in the current climates and contexts of research and the demand for certain types of knowledge and the endorsement of this in the development of evidence-based practice in Western neoliberal healthcare settings (Zeeman, Aranda, & Grant, 2014). Moreover, the current politics of healthcare research suggest serious ongoing challenges over the value and legitimacy of qualitative health research (Greenhalgh, 2016). Regardless of arguing qualitative research should be taken or is taken more seriously, having been incorporated into national health programmes of funding in healthcare research via the endorsement of mixed methods (Morse,

16   Kay Aranda

2012), others contest this, arguing that this version of qualitative research is reducing what are complex rich traditions to mere method. However there is an evident reluctance and retreat from funding more fully developed qualitative research studies, and hardly any interest in more theoretical, innovative, experimental or creative ways of thinking and knowing in health research; this is widely recognised globally, especially within neoliberal healthcare systems in rich income countries such as the UK, USA, Canada and Australia (Denzin, 2017; Lather, 2016; Fielding, 2017, Greenhalgh, 2016; Cheek, 2011). In this overtly positivistic world of funded healthcare research, qualitative research is reduced or narrows to approved methodologies or positivistic, scientific-outcome-based, realist qualitative and quantitative research, or systematic reviews, which are favoured over more creative, narrative, meta-ethnographic or critical reviews and syntheses (Dixon-Woods et al., 2006; Greenhalgh, Thorne, & Malterud, 2018; Savin-Baden & Howell Major, 2010).

Practices

Practices of qualitative research are in one sense the more explicit processes or tools of inquiry. The need to know how others have debated or argued and agreed how to design, conduct, implement and manage qualitative research are stages and practices essential for novice researchers. To fully appreciate these processes or practices means engaging with histories, controversies, unresolved dilemmas and the practices of improvisation, creativity and collaboration as well as engaging critically with a collective body of existing knowledge. Here various stages and tools regarding design, samples, practices over recruitment and access, or processes concerning how, for example, grounded theory or case study proceeds, stages of analysis, or issues of procedural ethics that blur into moral dilemmas over owning knowledge, and what confidentiality and anonymity mean arise. However, if practices are not merely tools or discrete events in an often-assumed linear approach to research, this collection shows how these processes and practices entail constant deliberation and thought. Moreover, if conceived as active forms of doing, as sets of practices comprised of decisions, competences, materials and meanings, then wider questions of the politics and philosophy of such come into view. Moreover, the policies, guides and protocols governing understandings of research processes and designs and or best practice appraisal tools, or evaluation and notions of quality in research, all become equally politicised practices; constituting forms of doing, measuring and categorising and embodying what is valued and what matters or counts (Gherardi, 2012).

Organization of the book

Debates over philosophies of humanism and posthumanism and of theories, politics and practices informing qualitative research are evident in all the contributing chapters, in varying mixes and degrees. The chapters are loosely positioned to reflect the vital and ongoing explicit and implicit dialogues with the continuum of philosophies of humanism and posthumanism. This allows for an appreciation of the deeply embedded humanist ways of knowing in qualitative research in healthcare that seek to uncover rich detailed theorised understandings and, for example, how posthuman is positioned, remains in dialogue with, and is always speaking to such central ideas, even when offering potential of different understandings or challenging the nature of such endeavours. All chapters share intentions to celebrate the richness of the full range of qualitative research used in healthcare and aim to always assess the value or usefulness of humanist and posthumanist philosophies, theories and the political consequences and practices from such thinking. The contributions are in part also ordered to best reflect the many ways criticality enters into qualitative research as previously suggested by Flick (2017), outlined on page 000 as a reminder. Though not exclusive for any one chapter, these levels of criticality are evident throughout the collection.

This will hopefully help you as readers to further consider the grounds from which qualitative research proceeds but also the intersecting or entangled nature of philosophies, practices and politics for your own research.

In the Chapter One, discussing research on crowds and crowd events, Chris Cocking starts with an exploration of philosophies, politics and practices by posing a provocative question of whether we do need to make explicit any philosophical grounds for our research. He explores in detail why and what happens to qualitative research when we do not. In his research he challenges taken for granted assumptions of crowds, as uncontrollable or chaotic, and given his topic, he argues the need to adopt a more practical or pragmatic approach to what might be contentious phenomena and where there may be disagreement in how crowds are perceived or portrayed. In doing so, he reveals how social pragmatism and interpretivist epistemology still imbue or underpin his work philosophically, but are far less relevant in making explicit. He goes on to show clearly just how key politics is, and how politically driven many of his decisions are, moving on to to offer an engaging, detailed reflexive account of his deliberations, rationales for certain practices or methods and the consequences of these positions and choices.

In discussing case study methodology, in Chapter Two, Kay de Vries shows how the complex intersections of philosophies, practices and politics underpin this evolving methodology. Now recognised as a flexible and pragmatic approach, she shows how case study has the potential to deconstruct and construct phenomena anew, and as viewed from multiple theoretical lenses. She offers details of the practices and politics of case study methodology, in its history, its approach, its strengths, as well as in the critiques of such. Case study methodology remains political in its aim to account for sociocultural political contexts, but there are always politics involved in deliberating over boundaries. In this methodology, it is what constitutes a case; often for practical reasons over feasibility and analytical potential, but of course this decides what becomes visible, what does not is, what is included or excluded, showing how this specific approach is used when working with people living with dementia. Philosophically, she shows how case study methodology, in its intention to be practical and flexible, does lean toward a realist or positivist perspective as it does have strong coherency with the ontology of social pragmatism and interpretive epistemology, but reminds us of the different scholars positioned along a continuum from realist to relativist and positivist to constructivist.

In Chapter Three, debating qualitative methods, the many choices, from familiar to novel and reimagined online and digital options, might seem relatively free of any philosophical or political considerations. However, in exploring these core elements of qualitative fieldwork, Julie Scholes critically explores these assumptions as she aims to discuss qualitative methods and revitalise debates by offering some 'strategic, creative and politically savvy suggestions'. She shows how dominant philosophies operate in current political contexts to devalue or diminish qualitative work to a detached method, devoid of methodological or theoretical considerations. However, she also wants to advocate for political acumen to convince funders, policy makers of the important contributions such insights can offer. Her chapter details best practices for interviews, focus groups, observation and documents, noting how shifting philosophies alter the nature of knowledge produced, as in postmodern approaches to observation. She illustrates her arguments with many rich examples from a range multidisciplinary work. In passionately advocating new approaches, offering practical advice, she argues for new alliances, evolving and resistant practices in the face of such politics, in order to develop convincing arguments, creative responses, fresh collaborations and plural perspectives.

In Chapter Four, exploring the many complex strategies and reflexivity that distinguish grounded theory from other qualitative methodologies and the experience of undertaking a grounded theory study, Julie Scholes shows how in doing so, there is always a need to explore history and the often fiercely contested debates and philosophical controversies over what is grounded theory and how it should proceed. This shows how historically contingent these different schools are, but also how political knowledge generation always is, and how necessary it is to be aware of histories, legacies and the resultant differing allegiances and how these impact on practices. As she argues, the omission, substitution and deletion of certain aspects of the grounded theory method, espoused by the different schools, are highly political acts, and it is where the politics of grounded theory is most controversial, contested and critiqued.

In her chapter on her journey as a doctoral student using grounded theory, Heather Baid (Chapter Five), engages fully with and details the many complex practices, politics and entanglements with theory and philosophy involved in developing a grounded theory. She shows how developing her philosophical position was a key transition point to her developing her project and the practices of grounded theory. Her contribution documents this journey detailing the many moments that require deep thought and critical reflexivity over questions of consistency, complementarity, and compatibility or justifying choices and positions with an example concerning dimensional analysis; here she shows how her politics, philosophical position shaped and justified her methodological choices. Using detailed illustrations as a means to share this learning, she shows how these choices and thinking were put into effect. In sharing these experiences and learning points gained from her PhD, she is also political in her intent to open up and expose and make explicit often hidden or tacit knowledge and experiences to collegiately support and help other postgraduate researchers.

In Chapter Six, in exploring phenomenology to practice and the related theoretical foundations and associated phenomenological methods, authors Kate Galvin, Oliver Thurlow and Rebecca Player discuss descriptive phenomenology especially, but also what sets phenomenology apart from other qualitative methods. In advocating a lifeworld approach as the grounds for inquiry, they further define a specific phenomenological approach and what this means in the pursuit of enquiry. They illustrate how specific phenomenological philosophies inform a phenomenological approach that translates into specific intents, practices or methods for carrying out empirical or applied research which aims to more deeply understand the phenomenon and its essential features. The importance of individual meaning-in-context is emphasised, but so too are the properties of significant phenomenon like dignity, loneliness, or wellbeing, that are recognisable to others in a shared lifeworld. They detail the many complex considerations, continuities and discontinuities between approaches and argue for an appreciation of the long and deep philosophical heritage of phenomenology in world of healthcare research that tends towards superficial uses of qualitative research; this is a political act.

Graham Stew (Chapter Seven), offers a further deep exploration of phenomenology and specifically debates questions of consciousness and experience. These questions span or can be positioned within the spectrum of humanism and post-humanism, with perhaps more leaning towards and in dialogue with post-humanism. However, not quite fitting, questioning boundaries, interestingly reveals the artefact of all our categorisations and conceptual dimensions as much of the material transcends this conceptual divide or relational qualities of humanism/posthumanism in its relationships to transpersonal psychology. He explores core categories and assumptions of consciousness, experience, and intentionality as both directed internally to thoughts and feeling and to external objects in phenomenology and reveals the philosophical complexity involved and the practical implications for qualitative research.

In exploring patient and public engagement and involvement for clinical commissioning in the NHS, in Chapter Eight, Debbie Hatfield shows how using different philosophically informed theories, spanning both humanist and posthuman principles, helped rethink the practices of ethnography and deepened political understandings of the role of materials in this sphere of work. She details the shifts in philosophical thinking or epistemic turns informing social theory to show the effects on questions of methodology or method. Offering an account of ethnography, she moves onto explore why ethnography is popular in healthcare research and as importantly, why a focused ethnography has emerged. She shows the invisible processes involved in patient and public involvement and engagement work, and the many elements that comprise these practices and forms of learning. Viewed differently, using different theoretical lenses based upon posthuman emphasis on the centrality of materials together with a social-contructionist approach of social learning theory, key properties of the sociomateriality of these practices emerge as entangled and constantly evolving.

20 Kay Aranda

In Chapter Nine, Alec Grant offers an engaging discussion of autoethnography, speaking to autoethnography in an autoethnographic way, and asking readers to consider this approach and its implications for qualitative research, in their own lives and in their own healthcare research. Philosophically explicitly informed by poststructuralism and later by posthuman insights, this contribution is a political call to engage with autoethnography knowledges in a complex spectrum of ways. He reminds us that autoethnographic writers testify to harrowing and cruel forms of social injustice of great cultural significance. In discussing the strengths or benefits and distinctive contributions, he equally reminds us of the emotional costs and politics of such work, in challenging conventional ways of doing research and in choosing to be positioned outside normative practices and conventions.

In Chapter Ten, Kay Aranda introduces feminist research and theory for qualitative researchers, but also argues for and explores further posthuman thinking as embodied in new materialist or material feminist theories and concepts. Arguing for the potential of these for healthcare research, she suggests this is even so when such thinking appears to challenge conventional understandings of the centrality of the human subject to our research endeavours, or notions of lived experience, agency or change. Hence, she especially reviews the implications of these ideas and thinking for popular qualitative health research approaches of narrative and participatory methodologies. With new materialisms or material feminism in more-than-human worlds being used to rethink health and wellbeing, mental health and recovery, stigma and disability, she discusses empirical examples and more fully the implications for qualitative methodologies and methods, as well as the limits involved in any uncritical turn to matter and materials.

Finally in Chapter Eleven, discussing what it means to be a reflexive auto-ethnographer, Alec Grant further challenges qualitative researchers to unpack or undo the concept of reflexivity to expose or reveal the politics, philosophies and practices involved. He shows how this may produce critical, ethico, strong and intersectional forms of reflexivity; he then moves on to suggest further potential with the posthuman concept of diffraction. In his own examples he shows how challenging norms are not without sanction, as in the discomfort of self-dialogue and of choices made and to come, or when writing about the dead and how this violates cultural ethical taboos. He argues for reflexive-diffractive auto-ethnographies in his quest to improve our worlds, and to offer multiple witness accounts of these worlds at particular points in time-space. This he argues is politically, even morally better than attempts to write *the truth*, irrespective of our qualified epistemological claims for knowing.

References

Agamben, G. (1998) *Homo sacer: sovereign power and bare life*. Trans. Daniel Heller-Roazen. Stanford, CA: Stanford University Press.

Ahmed, S. (2006) *Queer phenomenology: orientations, objects, others*. London: Duke University Press.

Andrews, M., Squires, C. and Tamboukou, M. (2013) *Doing narrative research* (2nd ed.). London: SAGE.

Aranda, K. (2018) *Feminist theories and concepts in healthcare: an introduction for qualitative research*. London: Palgrave Macmillan.

Barad, K. (2007) *Meeting the universe halfway: quantum physics and the entanglement of matter and meaning*. Durham and London: Duke University Press.

Benton, T. and Craib, I. (2001) *Philosophy of social science*. Basingstoke: Palgrave.

Beresford, P. (2013) *Beyond the usual suspects*. London: Shaping Our Lives Publications.

Boote, J. and Booth, A. (2015) '"Talking the talk or walking the walk?" A bibliometric review of the literature on public involvement in health research published between 1995 and 2000', *Health Expectations*, 18, 44–57.

Bourgeault, I., Dingwell, R. and De Vries, R. (eds.) (2010) *The SAGE handbook of qualitative methods in health research*. London: SAGE.

Braidotti, R. (2013) *The posthuman*. Cambridge: Polity.

Browne, K. and Nash, J.C. (eds.) (2010) *Queer methods and methodologies: intersecting queer theories and social science research*. Farnham: Ashgate.

Burawoy, M. (2015) 'Facing an unequal world', *Current Sociology*, 63(1), 5–34.

Butler, J. (2004a) *Undoing gender*. London: Routledge.

Butler, J. (2004b) *Precarious life: the powers of mourning and violence*. London: Verso.

Butler, J., Gambetti, Z. and Sabsay, L. (eds.) (2016) *Vulnerability in resistance*. Durham, NC: Duke University Press.

Butler, J. and Scott, J. (eds.) (1992) *Feminists theorise the political*. London: Routledge.

Charmaz, K. (2017) 'The power of constructivist grounded theory for critical inquiry', *Qualitative Inquiry*, 23(1), 34–45.

Cheek, J. (2011) 'Moving on: researching, surviving, and thriving in the evidence-saturated world of health care', *Qualitative Health Research*, 21(5), 696–703.

Crotty, M. (2003) *The foundations of social research: meaning and perspective in the research process*. London: SAGE.

Denzin, N.K. (2017) 'Critical qualitative inquiry'. *Qualitative Inquiry*, 23(1), 8–16. doi:10.1177/1077800416681864

Denzin, N.K. and Giardina, M. (2015) *Qualitative inquiry and the politics of research*. London: Routledge.

Denzin, N.K. and Lincoln, Y.S. (2018) *The SAGE handbook of qualitative research* (5th ed.). London: SAGE.

Dixon-Woods, M., Cavers, D., Agarwal, S., Annandale, E., Arthur, A. and Harvey, J. (2006) 'Conducting a critical interpretive synthesis of the literature on access to healthcare by vulnerable groups'. *BMC Medical Research Methodology*, 6(35), 1–13.

Dorling, D. (2015) *Injustice: why social inequality still persists*. Bristol: Policy Press.

Engelmann, P. (2009) *Badiou & Zizek: philosophy in the present*. Cambridge: Polity Press.

Falcón, S.M. (2016) 'Transnational feminism as a paradigm for decolonizing the practice of research: identifying feminist principles and methodology criteria for US-based scholars', *Frontiers: A Journal of Women Studies*, 37(1), 174–194.

Fielding, N. (2017) '"Challenging others" challenges: critical qualitative inquiry and the production of knowledge', *Qualitative Inquiry*, 23(1), 17–26. doi:10.1177/1077800416657104

Finlay, L. and Ballinger, C. (2006) *Qualitative research for allied health professionals: challenging choices*. Chichester: John Wiley.

Flax, J. (1990) 'Postmodernism and gender relations in feminist theory', in Nicholson, L. (ed.) *Feminism/postmodernism*. London:Routledge.

Flax, J. (1992) 'The end of innocence', in Butler, J. and Scott, W.J. (eds.) *Feminists theorise the political*. London: Routledge, pp. 445–463.

Flick, U. (2017) 'Challenges for a new critical qualitative inquiry: introduction to the special issue', *Qualitative Inquiry*, 23(1),3–7. doi:10.1177/1077800416655829

Foucault, M. (1974) *The archaeology of knowledge*. London:Tavistock.

Foucault, M. (1980) Gordon, C. (ed.), *Power/knowledge: selected interviews and other writings 1972–1977 by Michel Foucault*. Brighton: Harvester Press.

Galvin, K. and Todres, L. (2011) 'Research based empathetic knowledge for nursing: a translational strategy for disseminating phenomenological research findings to provide evidence for caring practice'. *International Journal of Nursing Studies*, 48, 522–530.

Gherardi, S. (2012) *How to conduct a practice-based study*. Cheltenham: Edward Elgar.

Gherardi, S. (2017) 'Sociomateriality in posthuman practice theory', in Hui, A., Schatzki, T. R. and Shove, E. (eds.) *The nexus of practices: connections, constellations, practitioners*. London: Routledge, pp. 38–51.

Green, J. and Thorogood, N. (2018) *Qualitative methods for health research* (4th ed.). London: SAGE.

Greenhalgh, T. (2016) 'An open letter to the BMJ editors on qualitative research', *British Medical Journal*, 352(563), 1–4.

Greenhalgh, T., Thorne, S. and Malterud, K. (2018) 'Time to challenge the spurious hierarchy of systematic over narrative reviews?', *European Journal of Clinical Investigation*, 48, 1–6. doi:10.1111/eci.12931

Hall, D.E., Jagose, A., Bebell, A. and Potter, S. (eds.) (2013) *The Routledge queer studies reader*. London: Routledge.

Haraway, J.D. (2008) *When species meet*. Minneapolis: University of Minnesota Press.

Hekman, S. (ed.) (1996) *Feminist interpretations of Michel Foucault*. University Park, PA: Penn State University Press.

Hesse-Biber, S. N. and Leavy, P. (2008) *Handbook of emergent methods*. London: SAGE.

Hill Collins, P. (2000) *Black feminist thought: knowledge, consciousness, and the politics of empowerment* (2nd ed.). London: Routledge.

Holloway, I. and Freshwater, D. (2007) *Narrative research in nursing*. Oxford: Blackwell.

Holloway, I. and Galvin, K. (2017)*Qualitative research in nursing and healthcare* (4th ed.). Oxford: Wiley Blackwell.

Honneth, A. (2007) *Disrespect: the normative foundations of critical theory*. Cambridge:Polity Press.

hooks, b. (1982) *Ain't I a woman: black women and feminism*. London: Pluto Press.

Hurwitz, B., Greenhalgh, T. and Skultans, V. (eds.) (2004) *Narrative research in health and illness*. Oxford: Blackwell.

Jackson, A.Y. and Mazzei, L.A. (2009)*Voice in qualitative inquiry: challenging conventional, interpretative and critical conceptions in qualitative research*. London:Routledge.

Jagose, A. (2009) 'Feminism's queer theory'. *Feminism and Psychology*, 19(2), 157–174.

Kovach, M. (2009) *Indigenous methodologies: characteristics, conversations and contexts*. Toronto, ON: University of Toronto Press.

Lather, P. (2016) 'Top ten+ list: (re)thinking ontology in (post)qualitative research', *Cultural Studies ↔ Critical Methodologies*, 16(2), 125–131.

Lather, P. and St Pierre, E.A. (2013) 'Post-qualitative research'. *International Journal of Qualitative Studies in Education*, 26(6), 629–633.

Latour, B. (2007) *Reassembling the social: an introduction to actor-network-theory*. Oxford: Oxford University Press.

Leavy, P. (2017) *Research design: quantitative, qualitative, mixed methods, arts-based and community-based participatory research approaches*. London: Guilford Press.

Lewis, R. and Mills, S. (eds.) (2003) *Feminist postcolonial theory: a reader*. Edinburgh: Edinburgh University Press.

Locock, L., Boylan, A., Snow, R. and Staniszewska, S. (2017) 'The power of symbolic capital in patient and public involvement in health research'. *Health Expectations*, 20, 836–844.

Lorde, A. (2007) *Sister outsider: essays & speeches by Audre Lorde*. Berkeley, CA: Crossing Press.

Lukes, S. (2005) *Power: a radical view* (2nd ed.). London: Red Globe Press.

Mason, J. and Dale, A. (eds.) (2011) *Understanding social research: thinking creatively about method*. London: SAGE.

Meeham, J. (1995) *Feminists read habermas: gendering the subject of discourse*. London: Routledge.

Mertens, D.M. (2007) 'Transformative paradigm: mixed methods and social justice', *Journal of Mixed Methods*, 1(3), 212–225.

Mohanty, C. T. (1988) 'Under western eyes: feminist scholarship and colonial discourses'. *Feminist Review*, 30, 61–88.

Morse, J.M. (2010) 'How different is qualitative health research from qualitative research? Do we have a subdiscipline?', *Qualitative Health Research*, 20(11), 1459–1468.

Morse, J.M. (2012) *Qualitative health research: creating a new discipline*. London: Routledge.

National Standards for Public Involvement in Research V1 (March2018) Available at: www.nihr.ac.uk/news/new-national-standards-launched-across-the-uk-to-improve-public-involvement-in-research/8141 [Accessed 28. 05. 19].

Nicholson, L. (ed.) (1990) *Feminism/postmodernism*. London: Routledge.

Palmer, V.J., Weavell, W., Callander, R., Piper, D., Richard, L., Maher, L., Boyd, H., Herrman, H., Furler, J., Gunn, J., Iedema, R. and Robert, G. (2018) 'The participatory zeitgeist: an explanatory theoretical model of change in an era of coproduction and codesign in healthcare improvement', *Medical Humanities*, 45(3),247–257. doi:10.1136/medhum-2017-011398

Piketty, T. (2014) *Capital in the twenty first century*. Cambridge, MA: President and Fellows of Harvard College.

Pope, C. and Mays, N. (2006) *Qualitative research in health care* (3rd ed.). Oxford: Blackwell.

Puig de la Bellacasa, M. (2017) *Matters of care: speculative ethics in more than human worlds*. Minneapolis: University of Minnesota Press.

Ranciere, J. (2010) *Dissensus: on politics and aesthetics*. London: Continuum International Publishing Group.

Ritchie, J., Lewis, J., McNaughton Nicholls, C. and Ormston, R. (2014) *Qualitative research practice: a guide for social science students and researchers* (2nd ed.). London: SAGE.

Rorty, R. (1999) *Philosophy and social hope*. London: Penguin.

Ryan-Flood, R. and Gill, R. (eds.) (2010) *Secrecy and silence in the research process: feminist reflections*. London:Routledge.

Scott, J.W. (1992) 'Experience', in Butler, J. and Scott, J. (eds.), *Feminists theorise the political*. London: Routledge.

Savin-Baden, M. and Howell Major, C. (2010) *New approaches to qualitative research: wisdom and uncertainty*. London: Routledge.

Schatzki, T.R. (2001) 'Introduction: practice theory', in Schatzki, T.R., Knorr Cetina, K. and von Savigny, E. (eds.), *The practice turn in contemporary theory*. London: Routledge, pp. 1–14.

Seidman, S. (2011) *Contested knowledge: social theory today* (4th ed.). Oxford: Blackwell.

Seidman, S. and Alexander, J.C. (eds.) (2001) *The new social theory reader*. London: Routledge.

Slutsky, J., Tumilty, E., Max, C., Lu, L., Tantivess, S., Curi, R., Whitty, J., Weale, A., Pearson, S., Tugenhardt, A., Wang, H., Staniszewska, S., Weerasuriya, K., Ahn, J. and Cubillos, L. (2016) 'Patterns of public participation: opportunity structures and mobilization from a cross-national perspective', *Journal of Health Organization and Management*, 30 (5), 751–768. doi:10.1108/JHOM-03-2016-0037

Smith, T.L. (2012) *Decolonising methodologies: research and indigenous people*. London: Zed Books.

St Pierre, E.A. (2009) 'Afterward: decentring voice in qualitative inquiry', in Jackson, A.Y. and Mazzei, L.A. (eds.), *Voice in qualitative inquiry: challenging conventional, interpretative and critical conceptions in qualitative research*. London: Routledge, pp. 221–236.

Taylor, B. and Francis, K. (2013) *Qualitative research in the health sciences: methodologies, methods and processes*. London: Routledge.

Turner, L., Short, N., Grant, A. and Adams, T. (eds.) (2018) *International perspectives on autoethnographic research and practice*. London: Routledge.

Watson, M. (2017) 'Placing power in practice theory,' in Hui, A., Schatzki, T.R. and Shove, E. (eds.) *The nexus of practices: connections, constellations, practitioners*. London: Routledge, pp. 169–182.

West, D. (2010) *Continental philosophy: an introduction* (2nd ed.). Cambridge: Polity.

Wilson, P., Mathie, E., Keenan, J., McNeilly, E., Goodman, C., Howe, A., Poland, I., Staniszewska, S., Kendall, S., Munday, D., Cowe, M. and Peckham, S. (2015) 'Research with patient and public involvement: a realist evaluation – the RAPPORT study. Available at: www.ncbi.nlm.nih.gov/pubmed/26378332 [Accessed 26. 05. 19]

Zeeman, L., Aranda, K. and Grant, A. (2014) *Queering health: critical challenges to health and healthcare*. Ross-on-Wye: PCCS.

1

QUALITATIVE RESEARCH AND IDEOLOGICAL PRAGMATISM?

Chris Cocking

Introduction

In this chapter I will look at the pragmatic approach that I have taken when conducting and disseminating the qualitative research I have done into crowd behaviour and collective resilience, and how I have incorporated this into my teaching methods. Over the years I feel I have become something of a poacher turned gamekeeper, as I have been on a journey that started as a crowd participant, but I have ended up as more of an observer. Either by accident or design, I have found myself in many different kinds of crowds (such as; political demonstrations; revolutions; music festivals; and sports events), and I always found there to be a mismatch between how myself and others around me experienced these events and how they were often portrayed afterwards. It confused and annoyed me in equal measure that what I found overall to be largely positive events were often portrayed by outside observers in much more negative ways. Through a series of fortuitous choices and happy coincidences, I have since found myself in the fortunate position where I have been able to develop my interest in crowds into a career pathway. Therefore, my academic career has been spent largely trying to rehabilitate crowds and debunk the myths that are so often presented about them in dominant discourse (e.g. that they are prone to irrational/ selfish behaviour, and that society should fear them because of the potential risk of 'contagion'[1] of any such 'irrational' behaviour), and this has sometimes led to light-hearted accusations that I could be described as the academic equivalent of an 'ambulance chaser' (when people are running away from crowds – I am the kind of person who runs towards them). Therefore, I am happy to declare openly my own positive bias

1 There is an ESRC funded project at the University of Sussex currently exploring the problems inherent in the contagion approach to social influence in crowds http://www. sussex.ac.uk/beyondcontagion/

26 Chris Cocking

towards crowds, and I frequently challenge the way in which crowd events tend to be portrayed in social and popular discourse via my blog 'Don't Panic!'.[2] I also feel proud to be part of a broader tradition within Social Psychology studying crowds that was inspired by the ground-breaking research done by Steve Reicher (1984) into the St Paul's riots in Bristol in the early 1980s and began the work of reclaiming our understanding of crowds away from previous irrationalist perspectives. His explicit aim to make crowds a safer place has inspired many researchers since, and has influenced the field of public order policing (Stott, 2009) and emergency planning and response (Drury, 2012, 2018).

However, despite this more positive view of crowds that myself and others involved in researching them have (which no doubt means that we could be accused of having preconceived and biased views of crowds), I have found that my own methodological approaches to studying crowds are often driven largely by pragmatic considerations, and this sometimes sets me apart from other researchers using similar methodologies. So, for instance, it can be more practical to study people's experiences of crowd events using qualitative approaches (such as interview and focus group studies), as it can be difficult giving out questionnaires in the middle of a riot![3] Therefore, I have not normally found it necessary to provide detailed epistemological and/or ontological explanations for my own choice of methodology – something that can conflict with the views of other proponents of qualitative methodological perspectives.

So, in this chapter I will explore how taking a pragmatic (and sometimes more systematic) approach to qualitative research may fit (or not) within broader qualitative research methodological paradigms and will consider the practicalities of conducting qualitative research without having an explicitly predefined ontological and/or epistemological position. Issues I will explore will include: the adoption of pragmatic approaches to research; the issue of bias in qualitative research; how I have reported my findings in a systematic and/or generalisable way for practitioners to use; the appropriateness (or not) of including reflexive discussions; and how I incorporate my own approaches to qualitative research methods into my teaching practice in a way that is useful for students wanting to conduct their own research using similar approaches.

Ideological pragmatism

Throughout my research career, I have tended to feel as an outsider – a position that I have accepted and perhaps sometimes even revelled in. The field of Social Psychology is often considered to be very positivist (this is sometimes even used as a term of abuse by qualitative researchers; Oakley, 2000), with an emphasis on

---

2   http://dontpaniccorrectingmythsaboutthecrowd.blogspot.co.uk/
3   It is of course possible to conduct post hoc quantitative research on crowd events, and Drury et al. (2015) did exactly this to explore experiences of a large outdoor concert held on Brighton beach in 2002.

hypothesis testing via experimental and/or correlational studies, and I have been to many a psychology conference where after spending a day listening to research presentations, one could be forgiven for thinking that human behaviour was governed solely by the results from 2 X 2 ANOVA[4] tables. I would often delight in telling people that I studied crowd behaviour and its implications for crowd safety management, as a common response I would get would be along the lines of 'Oh, that sounds very applied!', which I inferred as meaning that they felt my research was unusual for having an application in the real world. This sense of maverick status was further enhanced when I realised that my pragmatic choices for my research methodologies were also considered unusual by many in the field of qualitative research. This quickly became apparent to me when I first started teaching Qualitative Research Methods (QRM) to Master's students at the University of Brighton. So, for instance, I would often be asked by students during my teaching sessions what my ontological and/or epistemological position was, and when I replied that I didn't have one, this would often be met with puzzled looks as it clearly differed from what other colleagues had told them in other classes. I would even sometimes get asked by some of the more confident students, 'wouldn't your other colleagues involved in qualitative research call you a naïve realist?', to which I would be tempted to reply – 'not to my face, I hope they wouldn't!' However, my lack of a predefined methodological position didn't stem from a failure to engage with a sufficient body of literature, and I have always consciously felt that having too rigid an ideological approach to one's own choice of research methodology was potentially problematic, as there was a risk of fetishizing the research process over the content of the story that one wanted to tell. Therefore, I agree with Janesick's (2000) call to avoid 'methodolatry' which she termed as

> a pre-occupation with selecting and defending methods to the exclusion of the actual substance of the story being told. Methodolatry is the idolatry of method, or a slavish attachment and devotion to method, that so often overtakes the discourse.
>
> *(p. 390)*

Furthermore, others such as Holloway and Todres (2003) have argued against exclusivity of method, and that pragmatism within qualitative research should not be denounced out of hand, as the variety of possible approaches encourages a degree of flexibility:

---

4   ANOVA (analysis of variance) is a statistical technique used to compare multiple mean scores and is popular in quantitative social science research

28 Chris Cocking

> Precise definitions of specific qualitative approaches are still not settled and boundaries often blurred. We do not wish to advocate exclusivity or an elitist approach, nor do we see pragmatism as a 'methodological crime'.
>
> *(p. 355)*

So, my choices for using my own research methodology have often been influenced by a similar rejection of methodolatry and instead been guided by pragmatic considerations for data collection and analysis. For instance, my PhD was funded by the ESRC Global Environmental Change (GEC) Programme (that promoted multidisciplinary research in the UK social sciences from 1990–2000) and explored the psychological impact of climate change and how to promote more pro-environmental action by encouraging a greater sense of efficacy in individual and collective environmental actions. It involved comparative studies of the perceived efficacy of involvement in various pro-environmental behaviours and used a mixture of qualitative and quantitative research methods (such as interview and questionnaire studies).[5] One of the largest parts of my data collection was an ethnographic study of the direct-action protests against the construction of the A34 Newbury bypass 1996–1998.[6] My choice of ethnographic methodology to conduct this study was a pragmatic decision as I had come from the environmental protest scene myself and had been a research participant in John Drury's PhD study on the campaign against the M11 link road in East London in the early 1990s[7] (Drury, 1996). Therefore, I was aware that at the time there was a general distrust of the media (and even academics) among campaigners, due to the suspicion that they were not really interested in the underlying issues, and merely wanted to write their own story that did not necessarily present the protestors' values or aims accurately. Therefore, in order to find participants that would be willing to talk to me, I decided to get down and dirty and do an ethnographic study (also known as Participant Observation [PO]) of anti-roads protests, as I felt there was a greater chance that I would get participants to trust me and so be more open to sharing their experiences with me if I was actively involved in their campaign, as activists may question why they should help careerist academics whose commitment to the cause does not extend beyond their data collection period.

The psychology department at the University of Surrey (where I did my PhD) had a very positivist approach at the time, and so I often felt that my research was outside of most of my colleagues' own interests. I also expected that my methodology would be pulled apart at my Viva exam, so I devoted a significant portion of my methodology chapter to justify my use of ethnography, and was inspired by Sasha Roseneil's (1993) justification of her own ethnographic study of anti-war

---

5 See Cocking & Drury (2004) for an example of the quantitative data that were published.
6 https://en.wikipedia.org/wiki/Newbury_bypass
7 https://en.wikipedia.org/wiki/M11_link_road_protest

protests at Greenham Common air base in Berkshire in the 1980s (which is very close to where the Newbury bypass protests later happened):

> I . . . would not been able to interview most of the women I did, had I not been a Greenham Woman myself. Greenham was an extremely intense 'life-changing' experience which many of my interviewees said they would never have agreed to talk about to someone who had not shared it. . . . I am convinced that the degree of intimacy between myself and the women I interviewed was the product of our shared experiences and was only possible because they knew that I was a Greenham woman and a feminist first . . . and a sociologist second.
>
> *(p. 191)*

Fortunately, I was able to make the case at my Viva that my pragmatic choice of ethnographic methodology was justified given that my chosen participant group was potentially difficult to reach and engage with. Since I got my PhD in 1999 it seems to have become accepted that ethnographic research is a valid method of data collection in the Social Sciences, and such studies are now more common.

Bias?

Because my own approach to using qualitative methodology is quite pragmatic, I feel that it is freer of what I consider to be the philosophical and ideological baggage that underpins other qualitative approaches (other than that it shares the broader philosophical aim to focus on people's experience of phenomena that drives most qualitative research). However, I would never claim that my research is free from bias, and furthermore, I would argue that all academic research methods (both qualitative and quantitative) involve bias at some point, not least because one chooses the area to research that one has an interest in (and passion for), and so no form of research could be considered as value free. The bias I have in my research is there because I have spent my academic career trying to rehabilitate the crowd from the irrationalist perspectives that are so depressingly common in current social discourse. Furthermore, Reicher's (1996) account of how irrationalist perspectives of crowds have influenced right-wing demagogues throughout history, along with Stott's (2009) observation that they have also influenced public order policing tactics, highlight the clear need to reclaim our understanding of crowds from such ideological (and deeply flawed) perspectives. Therefore, I have a more positive view of the crowds I observe, as I am usually sympathetic to their aims and values, and my published work is usually an attempt to undo (or at least problematize) irrationalist interpretations of crowd behaviour. A notable exception to this is my observations of street demonstrations by the far-right English Defence League[8] and

8   https://dontpaniccorrectingmythsaboutthecrowd.blogspot.com/2013/09/variations-in-views-of-edl-protest-in.html

30 Chris Cocking

the March for England[9] during 2013–2014 (whose nationalistic and openly Islamophobic ideology I rejected completely).

Positive bias towards crowd events and their participants can be unavoidable when using ethnographic methods to explore crowd behaviour, since such behaviour often happens in a context of intergroup conflict, so conducting Participant Observation (PO) may involve having to take sides to gather data, and that such partisanship may even be necessary (Drury & Stott, 2001). This is because in order to be able to research those involved in crowd conflict (which can also entail involvement in illegal activity), a researcher usually needs to be accepted by the participants they intend to investigate, and openly sharing their aims and values is usually vital in building up such trust. As crowd conflict usually involves two or more groups in opposition with each other, building up such relationships of trust with one side, has the obvious disadvantage that trust from the group on the other side of the conflict will inevitably decrease. Therefore, conducting such ethnographic research usually results in only a partial view of the phenomenon in question, because it is usually more practical (and also potentially safer for the researcher) to attempt to collect data from only one side. However, it is also possible, that in trying to show evenhandedness and collect data from both sides, the researcher could become distrusted by both as they are talking to the 'enemy' (Wright, 1978). Furthermore, Drury and Stott (2001) argue that the unpredictability of crowd behaviour makes it ideally suited for exploration by PO because of its 'supremely opportunistic data-gathering framework' (p. 50). Therefore, such an opportunist approach to data collection can create a definite advantage in studying crowd behaviour, and when considering the subsequent stage of research (data analysis), there are equally pragmatic approaches that have also been useful in my research.

Thematic analysis – pragmatic building blocks

The pragmatic approach that I have taken to my own research means that I have also been drawn to more pragmatic forms of data analysis, and so it is perhaps no surprise that I have frequently used Thematic Analysis (TA) in my published research (e.g. Cocking, 2013a, 2013b; Cocking & Drury, 2004; Cocking et al., 2018). I have found TA a very useful method of analysis in its own right, but also as a first stage to get familiar with the data before using more detailed forms of analysis (such as Interpretative Phenomenological Analysis [IPA] or Discourse Analysis [DA]) which are covered in more detail later on in this chapter – a view endorsed by Braun and Clarke (2006):

9   https://dontpaniccorrectingmythsaboutthecrowd.blogspot.com/2014/04/the-ma rch-for-england-and-limits-of.html

It is the first qualitative method of analysis that researchers should learn, as it provides core skills that will be useful for conducting many other forms of qualitative analysis.

(p. 78)

Furthermore, because TA focuses largely on the practicalities of how to codify and analyse the data that one is presented with, it largely avoids getting drawn into the ideological debates that can attract other approaches, and is popular because of its flexibility:

> Thematic analysis… is not another qualitative method but a process that can be used with most, if not all, qualitative methods and that allows for the translation of qualitative information into quantitative data, if this is desired by the researcher.
>
> *(Boyatzis, 1998, p. 4)*

However, such flexibility could also become a disadvantage if the consistency of the analysis is then negatively impacted: 'While thematic analysis is flexible, this flexibility can lead to inconsistency and a lack of coherence when developing themes derived from the research data', (Holloway & Todres, 2003, p. 2)

Braun and Clarke (2006) argue that TA can be popular with novice researchers as it doesn't require the more detailed theoretical and technical knowledge often associated with other approaches (such as Grounded Theory or IPA), and Holloway and Todres (2003) argue that TA could even become part of later phenomenological approaches. However, a possible disadvantage is that because there is comparatively less written on TA than other research methodologies, this could then make it more difficult for novice researchers to do systematic and/or rigorous analysis of data as there is less published guidance:

> While much has been written about grounded theory, ethnography, and phenomenology, this trend has not yet reached thematic analysis. There is insufficient literature that outlines the pragmatic process for conducting trustworthy thematic analysis.
>
> *(Nowell et al., 2017, p. 2)*

This isn't to say that Thematic Analysis is devoid of any philosophical background, and Vaismoradi et al. (2013) suggested that TA has a realist/essentialist and constructionist, factist perspective which assumes that the data collected is a more or less accurate portrayal of 'reality' (p. 400). However, this does highlight a possible limitation with factist perspectives, in that when trying to analyse data collected about events that are either controversial, or have competing narratives, one must be careful not to reify datasets from the participants, and make the claim that they are an accurate version of 'reality' (a topic that I will return to later in this chapter).

32 Chris Cocking

With regard to possible bias in doing Thematic Analysis of PO studies, it is possible that a researcher may have a conscious (or unconscious) bias to code data about participants and their views in a more favourable way (Drury & Stott, 2001). There is also a risk of bias in self-reporting by participants who have been involved in crowd conflict with the police (Cocking, 2013a). Therefore, it is possible that both researcher and participants could harbour negative views of the police and their approach to managing crowd 'disorder' from their own experience of such crowd events (either as a participant or as an observer). However, my own research on crowd flight in disorder (Cocking, 2013b) has found that participants who experienced Police charges tended to report an increased sense of unity with fellow crowd members and an increased bias against the police after the charges, above and beyond of whether they were experienced political activists or not (and so would have presumably already have had an existing anti-police bias). There can also be possible self-reporting bias in crowd events that do not involve overt inter-group conflict, such as emergencies (Cocking 2013b), as survivors of mass emergencies may feel a self-presentational bias not to report behaviours that may present them in a bad light (e.g. if they behaved selfishly towards others). How-ever, concerns of such participant/ observer bias may be over-stated as data trian-gulation methods used in my own research (e.g. Drury et al., 2009b) has shown that selfish behaviour is quite rare overall in mass emergencies, and in any case accounts of others' selfish behaviour (which would not be susceptible to self-pre-sentation bias) tend to also be uncommon.

Reporting and dissemination of findings

I have come to realise that the ways in which one can present and disseminate one's research findings (and for whom it is produced) can vary with the academic culture in which one finds oneself. So, for instance, in my own published work, I have tended to provide systematic numerical accounts of the data sets that I col-lected and analysed (often including interview length, mean word count, inter-rater reliability of the coding system used, etc.). I had originally assumed that this was the norm, as I had had this approach drilled into me from when I first began doing qualitative research as it was common practice in the Psychology depart-ments at Surrey and Sussex where I began my research career. Such formats were also expected to appear in the papers we submitted to the peer-reviewed psy-chology journals (mainly those published by the British Psychological Society)[10] that one was under pressure to publish in, so that they could be included as high impact research outputs at the next Research Excellence Framework (REF)[11] – an exercise undertaken by UK higher education bodies to quantify and measure the supposed 'impact' of academic research and allocate funds accordingly. Therefore, I had somewhat naively assumed that this approach to research

10 https://www.bps.org.uk/publications/bps-journals
11 https://www.ref.ac.uk/

presentation was the norm. However, when I began teaching Qualitative Research Methods (QRM) at the University of Brighton, it dawned on me that such systematic approaches to research were not necessarily shared by all my peers, and that such an approach was even considered by some as falling into a positivist/realist trap that they so studiously avoided. This no doubt contributed to the confused faces I encountered in students when I first began teaching QRM, and I quickly learnt to pre-empt similar future responses by embedding into my teaching the notion that qualitative research is a broad church with a varied flock of adherents and believers, and that there are multiple different ways in which one's work can be reported.

Furthermore, I believe that the way I disseminate my findings also reflects my pragmatic approach to research, as I am very passionate about getting out of the ivory towers of academia and applying my work to solving real world problems. This passion has not gone unnoticed by others, and in a recent article for the online psychologist about the impacts that our academic research can have for emergency planning and response, I was described by the Principal Investigator (John Drury) on the ESRC project on mass emergencies that I worked on at Sussex University from 2004–2007 as 'impatient with academia and . . . more interested in producing knowledge that could be used'[12] (perhaps one of my favourite descriptions that others have made of me!). I am also in the fortunate position that while the importance of the impact of academic research has become something of a truism in recent years (and with it comes the implicit threat of reduced funding via the REF if the ability to show such impact is not forthcoming), there is a more obvious connection between research into crowd behaviour and real-world applications. This is because one can make a strong case that where current evidence-based models of crowds are implemented into the field of emergency planning and response, then this can help save lives. Furthermore, the 1989 Hillsborough football disaster is a tragic example of what can happen if current models of crowd behaviour are not followed, and event planning is considered from a coercive, crowd control perspective, rather than from a more facilitative, crowd management perspective (Cocking, 2014). Therefore, a significant proportion of my outputs are not just aimed at traditional academic sources (e.g. high-impact, peer-reviewed journals that focus on developing and defining abstract theoretical perspectives). Instead, I am also often asked to write short articles for applied and/or practitioner journals (see Cocking, 2018a, 2018b for two recent examples), present similar papers at practitioner conferences and/or exhibitions, and sometimes to advise on emergency planning guidelines and/or the physical infrastructure used to promote safe and efficient evacuations during emergencies. All these activities can help explain in lay terms the possible practical applications of my work for emergency planning and response to a wider audience of interested users beyond academia, including to practitioners, policy makers and the media. For example, work I have done on the concept of

12   https://thepsychologist.bps.org.uk/volume-29/february/riots-crowd-safety

34 Chris Cocking

zero-responders in emergencies (Cocking, 2013b) was recently cited within the 2018 Kerslake report into the Manchester Arena bombing (pp. 154–156),[13] and I am currently exploring the implications of Kerslake's recommendations for emergency planning and response (primarily that the potential role of zero-responders in emergencies needs to be considered within emergency response, and that there should be greater provision for first aid training amongst the general public).

Reflexivity (or not?)

Use of reflexivity is often popular (and sometimes expected) in health-related qualitative research, and there are certainly situations where it would be useful and appropriate to include the researcher's own views and relevant experiences (such as if they have had lived experience of a health condition that is the focus of the research). However, when writing about my own research into crowd behaviour, I don't tend to include reflective passages (and have not yet done so in my papers submitted for publication in academic journals). When I was a novice researcher in psychology, this was not something that had even occurred to me to do (and this could again probably be viewed as another facet of the positivist research culture from whence I emerged). So, it wasn't until I began teaching QRM at the University of Brighton that it occurred to me that one might be expected to include some reflection within one's writing, and I found myself being asked by students why I didn't include such reflexive accounts, as it appeared to be considered as standard practice among qualitative health researchers. This led me to think about why I didn't include my own reflections on my research into crowd behaviour and to consider whether I should start doing so. After some reflection, I concluded that this probably wouldn't normally be necessary and/or appropriate in my observations of crowd events (especially mass emergencies), as I felt that it would probably not significantly improve my ability to tell the particular story I wanted to relate, and that it could even deflect attention away from the experiences of those that mattered (e.g. those who had experienced the crowd events first hand). I feel that such a decision not to include my own reflections of crowd events in this way was justified – despite the irony of having found myself caught up unwittingly in major crowd events that became a future research focus for me on more than one occasion, and a source of some personal reflection, as I will now describe.

So, for instance, I had some limited personal experience of the 7/7 London bombings, having been in the tube system during rush hour on the morning of July 7, 2005 (I was evacuated from Waterloo East station at about 09.15, when the decision was made to close the Underground system). However, I was nowhere near any of the actual explosions, and so was ignorant at the time of the seriousness of the situation, and only found out later that morning via emerging media reports

13 https://www.kerslakearenareview.co.uk/media/1022/kerslake_arena_review_printed_final.pdf

what had happened and when central London went into lockdown. Therefore, I was very concerned that providing a reflective account within my published research on 7/7 could at best appear to be self-indulgent, and at worse I could have been accused of trying to colonise the traumatic experiences of others more directly affected by the explosions – something I wanted to avoid under all circumstances.

However, this isn't to say that my work is without any kind of reflection, and my web-log 'Don't Panic!'[14] often includes much more reflective accounts of my own research into crowd behaviour and how crowds are represented in wider social discourse. This blog was originally created because I was so incensed by the inaccurate and sensationalist media coverage of some major crowd events that I had recently experienced. I happened to be on holiday in Tunisia in January 2011 with my partner just as the Jasmine revolution was starting and witnessed a few demonstrations and riots before being evacuated by the Foreign Office after six days (but not before I had done multiple interviews with the UK media about the situation as word got round that a British crowd 'expert' was caught up in it). The media narratives of these events tended to focus on 'helpless' British tourists caught up in troubles in a foreign land that didn't concern them, and they seemed to buy very much into an uncritical irrationalist interpretation of crowds (that they should be feared and not explained), despite me saying otherwise while I was out there. This was particularly annoying, as I made a point during the media interviews that I conducted that neither myself or my partner felt threatened by crowd members during the demonstrations we witnessed, and at times we felt actively protected by them. So for instance, during one riot we got caught up in, we had to scatter through the back streets of the local town with the crowd when the Police arrived (there was a credible fear that they would open fire with live ammunition), and once the flight had stopped and we had time to pause for breath, a local woman came up to my partner and said in French 'you are Tunisian now, Sister' – which is probably one of my favourite examples of how a common identity can emerge from a shared experience of adversity![15] So, over time I have perhaps come to appreciate the potential utility of providing reflections on one's own research activities within the broader context of my work, but have not yet felt the need to do so within my published research outputs.

Embedding methodological pragmatism into the curriculum

In my own teaching practice, I tend to avoid providing an ideological background to the research methods I use, as I have found that using complex methodological terms can be quite alienating for novice researchers (even for students at Master's

---

14 http://dontpaniccorrectingmythsaboutthecrowd.blogspot.co.uk/
15 The concept of shared identities emerging from adverse experiences is a major theoretical tenet of the Social Identity Model of Collective Resilience (SIMCR) that was developed from our research into mass emergencies (Drury, 2012).

36 Chris Cocking

level). Instead, I try to provide a practical account of how I turned my own research from the raw interview data I collected into the final published version that emerges from the peer-review process and appears in print. This involves showing the students anonymised interview transcripts, the grids I used to organise the coded data, and the selected interview extracts and tables that appeared in the final Journal articles. I feel this helps illustrate in a practical way the process of data analysis that I went through, and the different possible ways that qualitative data that can be presented in published work. I have found that this 'nuts and bolts' approach often appeals to Master's students as they are often also starting their own research journeys, and seem to appreciate learning how they could organize and present their own research data. Furthermore, adopting this practical approach means that I seem to have avoided (at least so far!) attracting the accusations of solipsism in talking about one's own research that is commonly levelled at academics involved in undergraduate teaching.

What I have also found useful in my teaching is to explain how I went on a methodological journey to produce my paper on the 1989 Hillsborough football disaster (Cocking & Drury, 2014). My journey initially began by analysing the data using Thematic Analysis (TA), I later toyed with the idea of using Interpretative Phenomenological Analysis (IPA), and then finished up using Discourse Analysis (DA) – an approach that is popular in health and social care research (Morgan, 2010) to create the final written paper. In 2004–2005, I conducted interviews with four survivors of Hillsborough as part of a broader project into mass emergency behaviour that I was doing at the University of Sussex[16] (that was taking a critical view of the notion of mass 'panic'). I was struck how they all used spontaneously the term 'panic' during the interviews (and often before I had even had a chance to mention the word myself) to describe their experiences, so I wanted to explore these interviews in more detail than we did in our original Thematic Analysis of the overall interview study (Drury et al., 2009a). This was because I was mindful that attempts to explore the data relating to Hillsborough using the more basic approach to analysis that TA offered could have come into conflict with trying to maintain a factist perspective of providing an accurate portrayal of reality suggested by Sandelowski (2010) and Ten Have (2004) previously referred to in this chapter. Therefore, I decided to do a more detailed analysis of the data subset that consisted of the four Hillsborough interviews, using the coding we had developed from our Thematic Analysis as a starting point for more detailed analyses. I had initially wanted to use IPA as I though this could help me make sense of how participants made sense of their own experiences at Hillsborough, and that this might help explain why they used the term 'panic' so frequently in their accounts. However, I became increasingly aware that it was not going to help me illuminate the story I wanted to tell. This was because I wanted to critically pick apart the concept of panic, and explore why survivors of Hillsborough who would have had very good reason to reject the implications of the word 'panic', because using the term to

16 http://www.sussex.ac.uk/affiliates/panic/

describe their own and other Liverpool fans' behaviour could be interpreted that they were in some way responsible for the tragedy (something that the Hillsborough Independent Panel report[17] has since shown to be patently false), still used the term in their own discourse. So, over time and after detailed discussions with my co-author, I came round to the view that in order to critically explore the term 'panic', Critical Discourse Analysis (Fairclough, 2001) was better placed to do this than IPA (which takes a deliberately curious and non-judgmental approach to data analysis). This was because Discourse Analytic approaches can challenge 'common-sense' accounts of social reality (Willig, 2001, p. 107) using contentious terminology (such as 'panic'), and explore in more interrogative detail how and why survivors of disasters might use the term 'panic' to describe their experiences in diverse (and sometimes contradictory) ways. I felt that the resulting analysis using CDA provided a much better explanation of why the term 'panic' was so pervasive in participants' accounts – albeit with great variation in frequency and meaning and of usage. So, for instance, the term was used over 60 times in all four interviews, with one participant being responsible for over half of all mentions. The term was also used in multiple different ways to try and describe sometimes contradictory phenomena, including: fear, distress, loss of control, concern for others, and at least two participants explicitly rejected the notion of 'panic' in some way (such as denying that fans 'panicked').

An interesting question that I have been asked in my teaching sessions when explaining this methodological journey was whether I could be accused of influencing the results in a certain way to conform to my own bias to disprove the notion that 'panic' happened at Hillsborough. This was because an uncritical use of IPA to analyse participant's accounts could have concluded that because participants used the term 'panic' to make sense of their experiences, then this was then a 'real' phenomenon for them. I found that openly addressing this question (and encouraging students in future sessions to consider it, too) could then guide an interesting class discussion as to how qualitative research shouldn't necessarily attempt to seek the 'truth' about controversial events (and because the sample size for our study was only four participants, we were very careful not to make any claims about the generalizability of our findings) but that it was suitably placed to explore how people's accounts of such events could be constrained by social discourse, and also how they may resist such constraints (one participant explicitly stated 'the only way I can describe it as "panic"' [Cocking & Drury,, 2014, p. 94]), suggesting that he was aware of the limitations of the term). Using DA in our paper helped us overcome this apparent contradiction in participants' use of pathological language to describe events, and we explained this as follows:

> DA suggests that, while speakers may resist pathologiziation, their choices of words are constrained by what is culturally available. Therefore, this can

---

17 https://www.gov.uk/government/publications/the-report-of-the-hillsborough-indep endent-panel

38 Chris Cocking

explain why those who would reject attributions of their own pathology in mass emergencies may nevertheless use a term that implies a 'panicked' response to such disasters.

(Cocking & Drury, 2014, p. 88)

I tend to round up my teaching sessions by exploring how DA is frequently used in health and social care to challenge the dominant discourses that are often prevalent in organisations such as the NHS (Morgan, 2010), and also recommend to students that if they do choose to similar research using discourse analytic approaches, they probably don't use my timeline as a guide, as it took nine years from my initial data collection until the article finally appeared in print!

Conclusion

I hope that this chapter has helped describe my own approaches to qualitative research and how I include them within my teaching practice, as well as how they may differ from others' approaches (no doubt such divergences of views may very well be reflected within this very book!). However, I have always believed that the complexity of the human condition and how it is expressed requires different ways of exploring it and there should not be a one-size fits all approach. This is especially the case where one is looking at contentious phenomena where there may not be unanimity in how they are perceived and/or portrayed (such as crowd events). Furthermore, as our understanding of such contentious processes improves, changes in social policy and practice may become necessary to incorporate such advances in our understanding – something that has certainly happened in the study of crowd behaviour, and is a prime example of how a pragmatic approach to research can have direct practical implications. I think that understanding of such processes can also be easily included into the teaching curriculum, and could help provide a useful practical example for novice researchers at the start of their research careers, as they are looking for guidance on how they might go about taking the first steps on their own research journeys.

References

Braun, V. & Clarke, V. (2006) 'Using thematic analysis in psychology'. *Qualitative Research in Psychology*, 3, 77–101.

Boyatzis, R. (1998) *Transforming qualitative information: thematic analysis & code development.* London: SAGE.

Cocking, C. (2014) 'Hillsborough's lesson – don't fear the crowd'. *The Conversation*, 15/4/2014; https://theconversation.com/hillsboroughs-lesson-dont-fear-the-crowd-25618

CockingC. (2013a). 'Crowd flight during collective disorder – a momentary lapse of reason?' *Journal of Investigative Psychology & Offender Profiling*, 10(2), 219–236.

Cocking, C. (2013b). 'The role of "zero-responders" during 7/7: implications for the emergency services'. *International Journal of the Emergency Services*, 2(2), 79–93.

Cocking, C. (2018a) 'Zero-responders: a force multiplier?' *Crisis Response Journal*, 14(1). www.crisis-response.com/

Cocking, C. (2018b) 'Crowd management and behaviour in emergency situations'. *Building Control Journal*. www.rics.org/uk/news/journals/building-control-journal

Cocking, C. & Drury, J. (2004). 'Generalization of efficacy as a function of collective action and inter-group relations: involvement in an anti-roads struggle'. *Journal of Applied Social Psychology*, 34(2), 417–444.

Cocking, C. & Drury, J. (2014). 'Talking about Hillsborough: "panic" as discourse in survivors' accounts of the 1989 football stadium disaster'. *Journal of Community and Applied Social Psychology*, 24(2), 86–99.

Cocking, C., Aranda, K., Sherriff, N. & Zeeman, L. (2018) 'Exploring young people's emotional well-being and resilience in educational contexts: a resilient space?' *Health: An Interdisciplinary Journal for the Social Study of Health, Illness and Medicine*. http://journals.sa gepub.com/doi/10.1177/1363459318800162

Drury, J. (1996) 'Collective action and psychological change'. Unpublished PhD thesis, University of Exeter, UK.

Drury, J. (2012) 'Collective resilience in mass emergencies and disasters: a social identity model', in Jetten, J., Haslam, C. and Haslam, S.A. (eds.), *The social cure: identity, health and well-being*. Hove, UK: Psychology Press, pp. 195–215.

Drury, J. (2018) 'The role of social identity processes in mass emergency behaviour: an integrative review'. *European Review of Social Psychology*, 29(1), 38–81.

Drury, J. & Stott, C. (2001) 'Bias as a research strategy in participant observation: the case of intergroup conflict'. *Field Methods*, 13, 47–67.

Drury, J., Cocking, C. & Reicher, S. (2009a) 'Everyone for themselves? A comparative study of crowd solidarity among emergency survivors'. *British Journal of Social Psychology*, 48(pt. 3), 487–506. doi:10.1348/014466608X357893

Drury, J., Cocking, C. & Reicher, S. (2009b) 'The nature of collective 'resilience': survivor reactions to the July 7th (2005) London bombings'. *International Journal of Mass Emergencies and Disasters*, 27(1), 66–95.

Drury, J., Novelli, D. & Stott, C. (2015) 'Managing to avert disaster: collective resilience at an outdoor music event'. *European Journal of Social Psychology*, 45, 533–547.

Fairclough, N. (2001) 'The discourse of new labour: critical discourse analysis', in Wetherell, M., Taylor, S., & Yates, S. (eds.) *Discourse as data: a guide for analysis*. London: SAGE, pp. 229–266.

Holloway, I. & Todres, L. (2003) 'The status of method: flexibility, consistency and coherence'. *Qualitative Research*, 3, 345–357.

Janesick, V.J. (2000) 'Choreography of qualitative research design: minuets, improvisations, and crystallization', in Denzin, N.K. and Lincoln, Y.S. (eds.) *Handbook of qualitative research* (2nd ed.). Thousand Oaks, CA: SAGE, pp. 379–399.

Morgan, A. (2010) 'Discourse analysis: an overview for the neophyte researcher'. *Journal of Health and Social Care Improvement*, 5(1), 1–7.

Nowell, L.S., Norris, J.M., White, D.E. & Moules, N.J. (2017) 'Thematic analysis: striving to meet the trustworthiness criteria'. *International Journal of Qualitative Methods*, 16(1), 1–13.

Oakley, A. (2000) *Experiments in knowing: gender and method in the social sciences*. Cambridge: Polity Press.

Reicher, S. (1984) 'The St. Pauls' riot: an explanation of the limits of crowd action in terms of a social identity model'. *European Journal of Social Psychology*, 14(1), 1–21.

Reicher, S. (1996). 'The crowd century: reconciling practical success with theoretical failure'. *British Journal of Social Psychology*, 35, 535–553.

40 Chris Cocking

Roseneil, S. (1993) 'Greenham revisited: researching myself and my sisters', in Hobbs, D. & May, T. (eds.) *Interpreting the field: accounts of ethnography*. Oxford: Clarendon Press.

Sandelowski, M. (2010) 'What's in a name? Qualitative description revisited'. *Research in Nursing and Health*, 33, 77–84.

Stott, C.J. (2009) 'Crowd psychology and public order policing: an overview of scientific theory and evidence'. Submission to the HMIC Policing of Public Protest Review Team. Liverpool: University of Liverpool, UK.

Ten Have, P. (2004) *Understanding qualitative research and ethnomethodology*. London:SAGE.

Vaismoradi, M., Turunen, H. & Biondas, T. (2013) 'Content analysis and thematic analysis: implications for condusiting a qualitative descriptive study'. *Nursing and Health Sciences*, 15, 398–405.

Willig, C. (2001) *Introducing qualitative research in psychology: adventures in theory and method*. Buckingham: Open University Press.

Wright, S. (1978) *Crowds and riots: a study in social organization*. Beverly Hills, CA: SAGE.

2

CASE STUDY METHODOLOGY

Kay de Vries

Short history and background to Case Study methodology

Historically case studies were associated with medicine, psychology and sociology where cases were used to explore individual patients and social conditions such as poverty, immigration, and unemployment (Tellis, 1997a, 1997b). In the late 1960s and early 1970s, Case Study, as a distinctive research methodology, began to be used to understand the effects of both social and education programmes, using research techniques that relied on quantitative quasi-experimental and survey data. However, the results of these types of exploration failed to take into account the socio-political influences or the complexities of the programmes in practice, providing little evidence in support of, or change to, the particular programme. Education researchers, of the time, were challenged to broaden their thinking about research designed to evaluate and consider telling the story of the programme rather than discreet elements (Norris, 1990; Simons, 2009). Case Study is now recognised as a pragmatic, flexible research approach that facilitates researchers to explore their interest in the particular case thus enabling comprehensive and in-depth understanding of a varied range of issues across a number of disciplines (Hyett et al., 2014; Creswell, 2014).

As a qualitative research approach Case Study is considered particularly valuable when exploring contemporary phenomenon (the case) within its real-life context, particularly where the boundaries between phenomenon and context are not clearly visible (Baxter & Jack, 2008; Stake, 2008; Yin, 2014). Case Study is a methodology that supports deconstruction and reconstruction of certain phenomenon, viewed through a variety of theoretical lenses, allowing multiple aspects of the phenomenon, within the context, to be revealed and understood (Baxter & Jack, 2008). It is primarily used in the fields of the social sciences, psychology, sociology, and anthropology, but not exclusively; it is also used in economics and

42 Kay de Vries

in practice-oriented fields such as environmental studies, social work, education, and business studies. A Case Study approach permits description, exploration and understanding of phenomena in the context of the real world and allows researchers to explore the experiences of individuals or a collective (Anthony & Jack, 2009) with emphasis on intensively examining the setting and activities within that setting (Bryman, 2004).

It is generally understood that Case Study does not adhere to a fixed methodological, epistemological, or ontological position (Rosenberg & Yates, 2007). However, this approach can lean toward a realist or positivist perspective as it does have strong coherency with the ontology of social pragmatism and interpretive epistemology based on the different positions taken by the key methodologists (Creswell, 2014; Stake, 2008; Yin, 2014). For example, Yin's approach to Case Study is positivist/post-positivist (Lauckner et al., 2012) whereas Stake (1994, 1995, 2013) seeks out multiple perspectives endeavouring to collate diverse interpretations of a specific phenomenon. Stake's ontological belief is that reality is specific and unambiguously constructed and positions him in an interpretive/constructivist paradigm (Lauckner et al., 2012).

Different types of case study design

Cases can be single or multiple in scope (Yin, 2014); 'a case' can be: a single community, region or country; a single family; an organisation; an individual; or an event or incident; a study may be undertaken that considers multiple, similar 'cases', see examples of studies undertaken in the field of dementia care (Box 2.1).

BOX 2.1 EXAMPLES OF CASES IN RESEARCH ON DEMENTIA

Hospital sites across one country with the research focus on the organisational approaches to dementia care within each hospital. Each hospital comprised the 'case'.

A number of wards within the same hospital organisation focusing on the everyday practice of providing care for people with dementia. Each ward comprised the 'case'.

Ten individual people with dementia and their family member(s) (cases) experiences of admission on one hospital ward.

An in-depth study of one case; a person with dementia living at home, all persons (family members and significant others) that the person interacts with on a daily basis over a period of three months.

Case Study types have been categorised by a number of research methodologists. Both Merriam (1998) and Bassey (1999) were early educationalist researchers and categorised Case Study methodology as theory testing, storytelling, picture drawing and evaluative. Yin (1994, 2003, 2014) developed his approach to this methodology over time and identified three distinct elements. First that the scope of the study should be concerned with investigating a phenomenon in a real world context, particularly where the boundaries[1] between the phenomena and the context are not clear; secondly, that multiple sources of data need to converge in a triangulated[2] fashion; and thirdly, the case benefits from propositional[3] development to guide both data collection and analysis.

Stake (2008) identified three types of Case Study: 'intrinsic', which are undertaken to get a better understanding of a phenomenon; 'instrumental', which aim to provide insights into an issue through exploration; and 'collective', which extend instrumental to several cases, all of which are heuristic, rather than determinative. Categorisation of Case Study methodology by Simons (2009) proposes an ethnographic approach, with its origins in the fields of anthropology and sociology. This approach uses participant observation to achieve a close-up description of the context. It differs from traditional ethnographic methodology in that it can be conducted at different times in both familiar and unfamiliar cultures. Ethnographic methods, such as participant observation and interviewing, are used. In using these methods this type of Case Study focuses on both the instance in action, as described above, whilst also gaining insight into the socio-cultural context (Simons, 2009).

One of the strengths of Case Study methodology is that the method of inquiry aids the researcher to first identify the macro and then use the micro to defend and explore the theories chosen (Osbourne, 2005; as demonstrated in Box 2.2).

BOX 2.2 ETHNOGRAPHIC APPROACH

Ethnographic methods were used in a Case Study to capture the contextual conditions of practices in dementia care across three wards in a large hospital organisation. Observation data enabled the researchers to recognise and address the visibility of the socio-cultural context of everyday interactions with people with dementia within contemporary practice. Data were examined through theoretical lenses on the microstructure of interpersonal processes of care.

Stake (2000) stressed that true Case Study aims to learn as much as possible from the case. When studying human affairs, perception and understanding is gained when immersion in and holistic regard for the phenomenon is achieved. The case is not meant to be viewed as representative but as the context within which the phenomenon is observed and explored (Robson, 2004).

---

1 Boundaries are discussed later in the chapter.
2 Triangulation is discussed later in the chapter.
3 Propositions are discussed later in this chapter.

44 Kay de Vries

Developing and using a case study protocol

In keeping with most qualitative approaches to research Case Study methodology may be exploratory, descriptive, interpretive or explanatory and is well-suited to 'broad' and in particular 'how' (or 'in what way') research type questions (Cousin, 2009). Yin (2014) provides a useful five-step methodological protocol to guide researchers new to Case Study design:

1. Case Study question; the expectation is that a question is formulated following a thorough review of the relevant literature determining gaps in knowledge, or what is yet to be known about the problem under investigation. Case Study methodology starts with a curiosity about a particular case and asks what is going on in it (Cousin, 2009).
2. Objective criteria (or propositions)
3. The components that contribute to a case (establishing the boundaries to the case)
4. Logical linking of data to objective criteria/propositions
5. Criteria for interpreting the findings

Developing propositions

Case Study benefits from the development of propositions or objective criteria and theoretical concepts to guide data collection and analysis, which all contribute to trustworthiness, reliability and congruence (Amerson, 2011; Yin, 2014). Propositions are normally developed to help guide the research process and act much like hypotheses and offer statements of relationship. They direct the researchers' attention to something that should be examined and provide the rationale and direction for the data collection; they are the basis for initial data analysis and are supported or rejected during data analysis (Baxter & Jack, 2008; Yin, 1994, 2003, 2014). Propositions are taken from the literature and the researchers own perspectives of the concept and experience within the field (Box 2.3). They allow the researcher to link the data and relate it to the theory, thus initial pattern matching can commence (Yin, 1994, 2003, 2014).

BOX 2.3 EXAMPLE OF PROPOSITIONS FOR A STUDY ON DEMENTIA CARE IN HOSPITAL

Propositions – drawn from literature and practice observations and experiences of the researchers for a study of a number of wards within the same hospital organisation focusing on the everyday practice of providing care for people with dementia:

1. People with dementia are distressed and disorientated by the unfamiliar environment of an acute hospital ward.

2. People with dementia are not admitted to hospital because of their dementia, but generally as a result of an acute incident such as an infection or cardiac event.
3. Family members feel the need to be present to 'monitor' and 'support' care during the admission.
4. Staff in acute hospital have poor understanding of dementia symptoms.
5. Staff in acute hospitals are unfamiliar with providing care for people with dementia.
6. Acute hospital environments are not designed to support the needs of people with dementia.

The discourse in the literature about the use of propositions is far from clear. For example, Yin (2003) argues that propositions direct the researcher to aspects of the study that require examination as part of the whole study, and that the propositions are generally how and why questions and do not convey what should be examined but lay out what interests the researcher. However, it is claimed that propositions increase the manageability of the research and therefore likelihood of completion (Baxter & Jack, 2008).

Determining the unit of analysis and boundaries of the 'case'

The notion of boundaries and a bounded system are considered to be one of the hallmarks of Case Study methodology (Merriam, 2009; Stake, 1995; Yin, 2009). There is consensus in the literature on Case Study research about the need to define the bounded system and the components of each case (sometimes referred to as binding the case), with an established identity, that is 'the case' (or 'cases') making clear its analytical frame or object (Stake 1995, 2000; Thomas, 2010; Creswell, 2013, 2014; Yin, 1994, 2014). Cases are bound by geography, time and place, activity and place; or by definition and context; researchers collect detailed information, using multiple data collection procedures over a sustained period of time in the field (Creswell, 2014; Simons, 2009; Stake, 2008; Yin, 2014). The need for clear boundaries in case selection is important in order to ensure that the study is practically achievable (Baxter & Jack, 2008; Stake, 1995). Simons (2009) contends that it is wise to decide the boundaries of the case before the study commences but also identifies that there may be a need to refine the boundaries once in the field, to reflect any unintended shifts. These shifts could be politically influenced or simply undertaken because the researcher needed to re-conceptualise (Simons, 2009). Some case(s) may not have clear beginning and end points, and it is important to set boundaries that adequately bind the case(s) in time (Creswell, 2013). In many Case Study reports the researchers fail to adequately present their argument for the selection of the cases and the specified boundaries (Thomas, 2010).

Identifying the boundaries of the case is also essential to directing and managing data collection and analysis. This involves being selective and specific in identifying the parameters of the case including the participant(s), location, and processes to be explored, and establishing the timeframe for studying the case (Merriam, 2009; Stake, 2013; Yin, 2014) (see Box 2.4). This also includes establishing what the case will not be and helps to avoid the pitfall of attempting to answer a question that is too broad or having too many objectives.

BOX 2.4 EXAMPLES OF CASE BOUNDARIES

Hospital site as a case: each case was bounded by specific geography and demographics, i.e. hospitals were selected from a diverse range of sites to include areas of poverty, wealth, ethnic and cultural diversity, and rural and urban populations. Data collection focused on architecture design, strategies and policies related to dementia friendly environments and organisational management practices related to attention to people with dementia.

A number of wards within the same hospital organisation focusing on the everyday practice of providing care for people with dementia: the boundaries of the cases were determined by the environments and data collected: ward specialism; observation of the specific management and leadership styles practiced on a specific ward; observation of clinical and care associated practice; interviews with people with dementia, their families and with all staff who interacted with them; the use of an 'Approaches to Dementia Questionnaire' measure for staff; and relevant patient records and other documents pertinent to the care of people with dementia on each individual ward.

Ten individual people with dementia and their family member(s) (cases) experiences of admission on a hospital ward over a defined period: boundaries in this study included assessment scores of dementia using the *Mini-Mental State Examination* (MMSE), the *Cornell Scale for Depression in Dementia* (CSDD), the *Rating for Anxiety in Dementia* (RAID); patient medical records; the experiences of being a patient with dementia or a family member of that patient based on interview data.

An in-depth study of one case; a person with dementia living at home: The case boundaries were; a defined period of three months, multiple interviews with all persons that the person with dementia interacted with on a daily basis, observation of the environment and interactions, including interactions with pets, garden/plants, and any relevant objects/artefacts within the environment.

Triangulation

The term triangulation 'has been used, abused, and misinterpreted' (Denzin, 2012, p. 85) since it was first advocated in qualitative research. Denzin proposed that triangulation was not merely the combination of qualitative and quantitative methods but was the use of multiple forms of evidence to gain an in-depth understanding of the concept as each one yields a different picture and slice of reality (Denzin, 1970). A strength of Case Study research is triangulation, where multiple perceptions and a variety of procedures are utilised to clarify meaning and to identify the different ways phenomenon are perceived (Parahoo, 2006; Stake, 2008; Yin, 2014). Triangulation is also a validity strategy through which qualitative research methods can demonstrate credibility, confirmability and construct validity; established through the convergence of multiple sources of data to determine consistency of findings; studies that collect both qualitative and quantitative data neutralise the weaknesses inherent in each data type (Parahoo, 2006; Creswell, 2014).

Triangulation can be employed both at the study planning and design phase and in the analysis phase; in most research texts four main types of triangulation are described. These are: data triangulation, where multiple data sources are used which have similar foci but are used to obtain data from diverse groups about a topic and develop a full and rich description of the phenomenon under study (Gangeness & Yurkovich, 2006; Patton, 2002; Denzin, 1970). Method triangulation is the use of two or more research methods in one study (e.g. survey questionnaire, measurement scales, interviews, observation); investigator triangulation involves the use of two or more 'research-trained' investigators with divergent backgrounds to explore the same phenomenon; theory triangulation is where an assessment of the utility and power of competing theories or hypotheses are used deductively to examine data. Application of theory is considered essential when using Case Study methodology, as it is what connects ideas, explains patterns and holds the whole case together (Thomas, 2010). The selection of an appropriate theory through which to examine data does not have to ensue prior to commencing the study, although possible theories should be considered. Selection of theory usually occurs during data collection as ideas about 'what is going on' within the case begin to emerge. Theoretical literature relating to the topic should be explored throughout the life of the study, however. A fifth type, described by Parahoo (2006), is that of analysis triangulation, where the researchers use two or more approaches in the analysis of the same set of data. The benefits associated with triangulation are increased confidence in data, and a holistic and contextual portrayal of the phenomenon of interest. There is also the ability to present unique findings that may not be apparent when using one method of data collection; overcoming the scepticism associated with single method, single perspective and lone analyst studies (Patton, 2002). The effectiveness of triangulation rests on the assumption that the weakness in any particular method is redressed by other approaches (Silverman, 2013), and different sorts of data may also yield different results which can be both 'illuminative and important' (Patton, 2002, p. 556). See Box 2.5 for triangulation exemplars.

BOX 2.5 TRIANGULATION EXEMPLARS

Wards within the same hospital organisation focusing on the everyday practice of providing care for people with dementia: multiple data sources were used i. e. interviews, observations covering both day and night-time care; a questionnaire about attitudes to dementia, and examination of patient records; three investigators analysed the data; and data were examined through

48   Kay de Vries

> theoretical lenses, specifically the interpersonal processes of attachment theory
> and deception theory.
>
> Ten individual people with dementia and their family member(s) (cases)
> experiences of admission on one hospital ward over a defined period: multiple
> data sources included; assessment measures (as described in Box 2.4 pre-
> viously), examination of medical records, individual and group interviews, two
> investigators analysed data, and interpersonal process theories were applied to
> the data.

Data collection

Data collection spans a wide range of methods that include: interviewing; field
observation; focus groups; physical artefacts such as photographs and videos or film;
archival records; documents, such as meeting minutes, key organisation policy
documents; using questionnaires and surveying populations; undertaking activity
measures, for example cognitive measure of individual cases in dementia research.
Details on these data collections methods are not addressed in this chapter, however it is important to be mindful that when using Case Study methodology, a *huge*
amount of data may be collected. Consequentially the importance of maintaining
research journals and logs to keep track of methodological, observational and theoretical field notes during data collection; establishing a case study data base; and
keeping data organised is emphasised.

Criteria for analysing and interpreting data

Case Study analysis is a dynamic process that should occur throughout data collection and develop as the data is critically reflected upon. Continuing concurrent
examination of literature during data collection and analysis and write up is a
crucial feature of this process. The approach implies the research design can
remain flexible throughout the data collection period. However, there is no
definitive template to using Case Study methodology in presentation of the
findings but there needs to be a description of a case so that its nature is transparent to the reader. The analysis moves between the field and literature, this
maintains the reliability of the endeavour as it is a more naturalistic approach and
reflects the holistic nature of the phenomenon (Stake, 1994, 2013; Yin, 1994,
2009).

Stake (2013) and Yin (2009) both have systematic procedures for analysis
when using Case Study methodology. Yin (1994, 2009) stresses that any analysis will depend on the investigators own style of thinking and argues that
coding the data into numerical form or tabulation detracts from the holistic
nature of the data. Pattern matching and explanation building are the two
dominant analytical techniques in case study as they aid the reliability of the

findings (Yin, 1994). Pattern matching has been compared with the generation of themes where the researcher analyses the data looking for phrases and themes that relate to the propositions. Other methodologists support developing a more intuitive, affective, hermeneutic and imaginative approach to analysis and highlight how artistic forms, such as story boards, can help with interpretation of the disparate elements of the case and can lead to holistic insights (Simons, 2009; Thomas, 2010).

Generally, Case Study methodology is used to determine what is common and particular to the case, but it also highlights the prevailing uniqueness to each case. The individuality of the case is founded on the nature of the case, its distinctive history, the physical setting, and contextual influences such as, politics, culture and economics (Stake, 1994). To study the case fully a researcher may choose to gather data on all or some of the characteristics of the case as described above. Given the practical logistics of conducting research it is ultimately the researcher who will determine how long and what characteristics of the case need to be explored (Silverman, 2013; Simons, 2009). Stake (1994) argues that the individuality of the case is not universally appreciated and argues that there is a preference for theoretical development and generalisation that fails to acknowledge the value of the particular.

There are multiple ways in which a case can be reported. Case(s) may be presented as a journey, a narrative or story following a timeline, themed or categorised, or pattern mapped. It is important that the researcher(s) display sufficient evidence from data, providing as much detail of the case(s) as possible so that the reader may draw their own conclusions from the evidence presented. For example, Stake recommends presenting cases as vignettes or a brief descriptive story using episodes to illustrate aspects of the case to provide the reader with a 'story' they can recognise.

Multiple cases and cross-case analysis

Choosing multiple cases may be a challenge; for example, researchers need to decide how many cases are sufficient (Creswell, 2013). The number and type of case studies depends upon the purpose of the inquiry (Stake 1995). More than one case can potentially dilute the findings and provide less detail or depth of analysis. The benefit of multiple cases is that they add to the robustness of the study, and cross-case data triangulation, that is data convergence, adds strength to the findings, as the various strands of data are braided together to promote a greater understanding of the case(s) (Baxter & Jack, 2008). However, the process of undertaking cross-case analysis is not well documented (Yin, 2003). When a cross-case analysis is presented in the published literature it routinely presents the similarities or difference in emergent themes and little else (Creswell, 2013). Cross-case analysis is an area of Case Study methodology that is still evolving. See Box 2.6 for example.

50   Kay de Vries

BOX 2.6 EXAMPLE OF PRESENTATION OF MULTIPLE CASES AND CROSS-CASE ANALYSIS

A number of wards within the same hospital organisation focusing on the everyday practice of providing care for people with dementia. Each ward comprised the 'case'. The findings were presented in two sections (for a thesis this could be two findings chapters). In the first section/chapter an ethnographic description of each of the three different wards was developed that addressed the individual layout; the ambiance; the culture of practice towards people with dementia; the skill mix; etc. These were presented as a 'story' that revealed the culture in regard to dementia care practices on each of the individual wards. The second section/chapter (cross-case findings) involved re-examination of the data (using the 'story') and a combined process of thematic analysis and application to the data of the theoretical lenses of attachment theory and deception theory, in regard to the interpersonal processes of caring for people with dementia. Attachment theory allowed an understanding of the insecurity experienced by people with dementia when placed in an unfamiliar and frightening environment and how they sought to find security and safety through various forms of attachment; deception theory offered a lens in which to understand coercion practices used by staff to provide clinical care of people with dementia.

Critiques of Case Study methodology

The primary limitation of Case Study research is that it is relatively new as a research method Creswell (2014) and Anthony and Jack (2009) advise that Case Study is weaker or less rigorous than other methods. It is 'one of the most challenging of all social science endeavours' (Yin, 2014, p. 3); it is not only a linear process, it is also an iterative process that generates rich data rather than simplistic results, making all case studies unique (Yin, 2014).

Critics of Case Study argue that small cases cannot be generalised and the findings from such studies lack reliability (Tellis, 1997a, 1997b). Some authors also question whether Case Study can be classified as a methodology (Meyer, 2001; Luck et al., 2006; Flyvbjerg, 2006; Thomas, 2010). Hyett et al. (2014) critically analysed the methodological approaches of 34 published research projects using Case Study methodology. Their findings highlight that the flexibility of Case Study design is a liability and can result in 'haphazard reporting' therefore affecting the credibility of Case Study as a rigorous qualitative research approach (Hyett et al., 2014, p. 10). However, Rolls (2013) emphasises that just because these types of studies can be uniquely bespoke and don't necessary lend themselves to replication it doesn't invalidate them, and some of the most significant advances in psychology have come from one-off case studies. A further criticism of Case Study research is that it may be biased because the case is chosen to reflect the phenomenon (Yin,

1994; O'Leary, 2004; Tellis, 1997a, 1997b). The researcher, through their interest in the case, is at risk of expecting; even knowing that certain events, problems, and relationships will be important (Stake, 2000).

Chapter summary

Case Study is a pragmatic and flexible research approach that can be used to investigate simple through to very complex situations. It is also an approach that enables development of comprehensive understanding of a diverse range of issues across many disciplines including health and social science, environmental studies, social work, education, and business studies. Case Study methodology can be used to develop theory, evaluate programmes, and interventions. A wide variety of data sources and data collection methods can be used. It is a fitting methodology for both students and large research teams. Case Study has its own very specific design, data collection, and analytic procedures, however it is still an evolving methodology.

References

Amerson, R. (2011). 'Making a case for the case study method'. *Journal of Nursing Education*, 50(8), 427–428. doi:10.3928/01484834-20110719-01

Anthony, S., & Jack, S. (2009). 'Qualitative case study methodology in nursing research: An integrative review'. *Journal of Advanced Nursing*, 65(6), 1171–1181. doi:10.1111/j.1365-2648.2009.04998.x

Bassey, M. (1999). *Case study research in educational settings*. Buckingham: Open University Press.

Baxter, P., & Jack, S. (2008). 'Qualitative case study methodology: Study design and implementation for novice researchers'. *The Qualitative Report*, 13(4), 544–559.

Bryman, A. (2004). *Social research methods* (2nd ed.). Oxford: Oxford University Press.

Cousin, G. (2009). *Researching learning in higher education*. New York: Routledge.

Creswell, J.W. (2013). *Qualitative inquiry and research design: Choosing among five approaches* (3rd ed.). London:SAGE.

Creswell, J.W. (2014). *Research design: Qualitative, quantitative, and mixed methods approaches* (4th ed.). London: SAGE.

Denzin, N.K. (1970). *The research act: A theoretical introduction to sociological methods*. New Brunswick, NJ: Transaction.

Denzin, N.K. (2012). 'Triangulation 2.0'. *Journal of Mixed Methods Research*, 6(2), 80–88. doi:10.1177/1558689812437186

Flyvbjerg, B. (2006). 'Five misunderstandings about case-study research'. *Qualitative Inquiry*, 12(2), 219–245. https://doi.org/10.1177/1077800405284363

Gangeness, J.E., & Yurkovich, E. (2006). 'Revisiting case study as a nursing research design'. *Nurse Researcher*, 13(4), 7–18.

Hyett, N., Kenny, A., & Dickson-Swift, V. (2014). 'Methodology or method? A critical review of qualitative case study reports'. *International Journal of Qualitative Studies on Health and Well-being*, 9. doi:10.3402/qhw.v9.23606

Lauckner, H., Paterson, M., & Krupa, T. (2012). 'Using constructivist case study methodology to understand community development processes: Proposed methodological

52 Kay de Vries

questions to guide the research process'. *The Qualitative Report*, 17(13), 1–22. https://nsu works.nova.edu/tqr/vol17/iss13/1

Luck, L., Jackson, D., & Usher, K. (2006). 'Case study: A bridge across the paradigms'. *Nursing Inquiry*, 13(2), 103–109. doi:10.1111/j.1440-1800.2006.00309.x

Merriam, S.B. (1998). *Case study research in education: A qualitative approach.* San Francisco, CA: Jossey-Bass.

Merriam, S.B. (2009). *Qualitative research: A guide to design and implementation* (3rd ed.). San Francisco, CA: John Wiley & Sons.

Meyer, C.B. (2001). 'A case in case study methodology'. *Field Methods*, 13(4), 329–352.

Norris, N. (1990). *Understanding educational evaluation.* London: Kogan Page.

O'Leary, Z. (2004). *The essential guide to doing research.* London:SAGE.

OsbourneJ.D. (2005). 'Converting data to information for case study analysis: Decision services'. *The Journal of Innovative Education*, 3(1), 137–141.

Patton, M.Q. (2002). *Qualitative research and evaluation methods.* London: SAGE.

Parahoo, K. (2006). *Nursing research: Principles, process and issues* (2nd ed.). Basingstoke: Palgrave Macmilllan.

Robson, C. (2004). *Real world research* (2nd ed.). Malden, MA: Blackwell.

Rolls, G. (2013). *Classic case studies in psychology*(2nd ed.). New York: Routledge.

Rosenberg, J.P., & Yates, P.M. (2007). 'Schematic representation of case study research designs'. *Journal of Advanced Nursing*, 60(4), 447–452. doi:10.1111/j.1365-2648.2007.04385.x

Silverman, D. (2013). *Doing qualitative research: A practical handbook* (3rd ed.). Los Angeles: SAGE.

Simons, H. (2009). *Case study research in practice.* London: SAGE.

Stake, R.E. (1994). Case studies. In N. K. Denzin & Y. S. Lincoln (eds.), *The handbook of qualitative research.* Thousand Oaks, CA: SAGE, pp. 236–247.

Stake, R.E. (1995). *The art of case study research.* London: SAGE.

Stake, R.E. (2000). Case studies. In N.K. Denzin, & Y.S. Lincoln (eds.), *Handbook of qualitative research* (2nd ed.). Thousand Oaks, CA: SAGE, pp. 435–453.

Stake, R.E. (2008). Qualitative case studies. In N.K. Denzin & Y.S. Lincoln (eds.), *Strategies of Qualitative Inquiry* (3rd ed.). London: SAGE, pp. 119–149.

Stake, R.E. (2013). *Multiple case study analysis.* New York: Guilford Press.

Tellis, W.M. (1997a). 'Application of a case study methodology'. *The Qualitative Report*, 3(3), 1–19. https://nsuworks.nova.edu/tqr/vol3/iss3/1

Tellis, W.M. (1997b). 'Introduction to case study'. *The Qualitative Report*, 3(2), 1–14. http s://nsuworks.nova.edu/tqr/vol3/iss2/4

Thomas, G. (2010). 'Doing case study: Abduction not induction, phronesis not theory'. *Qualitative Inquiry*, 16(7), 575–582.

Yin, R.K. (1994). *Case study research: Design and methods.* Thousand Oaks, CA: SAGE.

Yin, R.K. (2003). *Case study research: Design and methods* (3rd ed.). Thousand Oaks, CA: SAGE.

Yin, R.K. (2009). *Case study research: design and methods* (4th ed.). London: SAGE.

Yin, R.K. (2014). *Case study research: Designs and methods* (5th ed.). London: SAGE.

3

QUALITATIVE METHODS

Challenges and celebrations of fieldwork in the health care setting

Julie Scholes

Introduction to qualitative methods

The chosen research methods used should answer the research question. However, what constitutes a valid, contemporary research question might be contested and, as a consequence, the merits associated with the impact of the subsequent research outputs. Research is inherently political, value laden (even if the value is to ensure absolute objectivity and a quest for truth) and potentially divisive. Research can be part of social engineering: i.e. what research gets funded by whom, but also what research gets reported, how, when and where and the extent to which that captures both professional and public attention (impact) and latterly that involves the public (for example, United Kingdom Clinical Research Collaboration [UK CRC], 2019). The quest for value for money particularly where public funds are involved, is both driven and drives policy but that can foreclose on what new knowledge emerges.

Health care research can transform society and public health through medical knowledge, technological discovery and understanding of the natural world. The UKCRC was established to coordinate collaboration, direct investment to patient priorities but what research is undertaken, by whom, can limit what is known, despite these best intentions. Funders invest in research and researchers they want (i.e. the topic is known, tried and tested, peer reviewed and the researchers have reputation in the field and professional esteem). Researchers work in very specialist fields therefore, what (and who) gets funded tends to follow ever increasing, specific avenues in greater depth, of larger sample sizes, seeking the single truth in answer to a very specific question. Careers are made on the back of it. Universities thrive on the outputs. Funding follows funding and universities are constantly seeking funding. Researchers have to be strategic to pursue research topics and deploy methods that will be rewarded with financial income but will also promise impact. Determining a topic and building a reputation in the field requires considerable luck as well as good judgement. Academic freedom is therefore limited but strict rules and boundaries can be overcome by dedication, industry and success. To circumnavigate the politics of research and become successful requires strategic foresight, creativity and steely determination. Entrée may be through working in multi-disciplinary teams, contributing to research based on mixed method, creating collaborations with colleagues based in clinical practice as well as those from academic environments, engaging public involvement, navigating and gaining approval from authorities that are established to facilitate health care research and involving patients (e.g. National Institute for Health Research [NIHR] – Research Design Service and Clinical Research Network Coordinating Centres). Building allegiances and contributing to science (and firmly *placing* public and patient involvement (PPI) centre of the research activity). *Representing* the patient and public voice *in* the research seems to be the way that qualitative data is represented in contemporary health care research.

Set in this context, the discussion on qualitative methods that follows, seeks to offer some strategic, creative and politically savvy suggestions. The aim is to raise the value of qualitative data beyond the illustrative example, case report or notional quote. A wise recommendation would be to become a Jill (or Jack) of all research trades, competent in all methods. However, that does not negate the necessity to build *expertise* in conducting field research (qualitative methods) in the real world (complex, challenging, dynamic), with patients who might well be vulnerable, enduring chronic ill health or suffering from the acute assault of illness, trauma or compromise. This overturns the myth that qualitative methods are chosen by people who can't do mathematics or don't like science. It is not an easy, intuitive option. It requires significant training, support, guidance, reflexivity and a relational ethic. As indicated, it might well require business acumen, a keen opportunistic eye and creative lateral thinking to build new collaborations with colleagues from other disciplines to answer research questions (most likely set by funders and policy makers) in a creative way that allows for new knowledge and fresh solutions to emerge.

The practice of interviewing

Interviewing is widely deployed by qualitative researchers (Flick, 2018). The approach to interviewing is governed by the epistemological, theoretical framework and methodology deployed to answer the research question. Therefore, there is no single approach to interviewing, nor where and when interviews should be placed within a research design. Instead there should be a sound rationale, clear purpose and justification for the way and how the interview is to be conducted.

Health care interviews involve people talking about their health, or as Kvale describes it: 'a conversation with a research purpose' (Kvale, 1996, p. 5). The purpose is that of the researcher(s)/commissioner(s). The participant volunteers their time and access to their private world, however limited that may be. Therefore, the practice of interviewing, particularly related to subjects of health and wellbeing, should inherently be an ethical act. The researcher has to consciously attend to NOT crossing the line to intrusion of private affairs and take care not to disclose private facts that can be attributed back to the interviewee (unless there has been prior consent to do so). These are the prima facie concerns of the researcher and made explicit in an ethics application. The independent ethic committee's role is to guard the best interests of the public. This is why the committee will ask for detail to assess that the questions asked at interview square with the participant information sheet and all elements of the consent procedure. The ethics committee will also want assurance that the interviewer is competent to undertake interviewing to produce data that is worthwhile and informative, compliant with data protection, and assurance of the way in which data will be presented and how confidentiality (and limits to confidentiality) will be handled. Therefore, from research design to the final report, the interviewer has to be consciously attending, noticing and acting to practice impeccably.

Interviewing is a skilled craft (Brinkman & Kvale, 2018); like all skills, it requires practice and experience to build expertise. Preparation is key to enable the practice of interviewing to flow, facilitate and explore the experience of the interviewee whilst attending to the practical and ethical issues that set that interview in context (Herbert & Rubin, 2013). Interviewing demands uncommonly common sense alongside a wealth of practical know how grounded in the epistemological and theoretical frameworks in which the research is framed. Indeed, however experienced a researcher might be, Janesick (2016) recommends that the researcher rehearse[1] their skills prior to entering the field and that includes revisiting the following: active listening, the praxis of ethical respect for the interviewee, skilled engagement with the participant, knowing one's role, putting the person at ease without overstepping boundaries, all whilst being aware of time, place and purpose. Like driving, the novice may struggle to assimilate all these layers and complexities associated with interviewing and that is why learning about interviewing, putting theory into practice and rehearsing those skills is so important. Of note, training exercises, simulation and rehearsal should not be confused with 'piloting interview questions'.[2]

---

1 Using the metaphor of dance to emphasise the importance of stretching before exercising to avoid injury, Janesick (2016) encourages researchers using qualitative methods to undertake a series of activities to warm up, tune in and attend to the detail of the interviewing procedure.
2 Piloting questions should be consistent with the methodology proposed and not inconsistent with the epistemological and ontological declarations made elsewhere in the research proposal or report.

56 Julie Scholes

BOX 3.1 PRAGMATIC CHECKLIST WHEN DECIDING THE INTERVIEW LOCATION

- Does the location compromise the integrity and privacy of the individual?
- Is it readily accessible, easy to locate by public transport?
- Is it appropriate to interview someone in their own home? Does this place an additional burden on the individual? Is it safe for the researcher to be alone with the interviewee? Has the interviewer invoked the Home Worker Policy and have all appropriate governance issues addressed?[3]
- Does the vulnerability of the interviewee suggest a need to hold the interview in a neutral location? Is it advisable that the location can offer immediate assistance and support should this be necessary (e.g. to manage distress, illness, fatigue)?
- The room at the location: is this appropriate, comfortable affording sufficient privacy and access to facilities?
- Can you control the room temperature, external/internal noise, sunlight in the room? Can you move the furniture to facilitate the interview environment? Can you provide refreshments? Have you checked the recorder and microphone alinement to ensure that you get a good recording (once consent has been obtained)?

Before the interview

It is good practice to phone, text or email the interviewee the day before to confirm that the arrangement is still convenient. This is of course contingent on having these contact details provided by the interviewee alongside their preferred medium for contact. After the interview, this medium can be used to thank the participant for their time and contribution.

Most research is undertaken alongside other commitments. Therefore, the interviewer needs to bring themselves to the research, the interview and role as interviewer. This might well require a different pace, a different energy. If possible, always allow one hour to set up the room, review the interview agenda/questions, check the recorder, location signage, do not disturb, phone off, etc. (See Box 3.1 for an interview location checklist.) Dependent on methodology you may need to revisit past interviews, analytical memos and pursue theoretical ideas emerging from data collected.

When organising interviews, ensure sufficient time is made available to write a hot reflective note about the experience, what has been learnt from the interview and what further action needs to be addressed as a consequence of that new insight, before you expect the next interviewee. Also ensure no crowding or overlap between participants especially if the subject is sensitive or individuals would not like to be seen by others. Using public transport can give you that space and time

---

3 This will include gaining appropriate background checks, including disclosure and barring DBS, occupational health checks, assessment of research competence and, if required, an Honorary Contract (NIHR Research Passport, 2019).

to cool yourself out through this reflective writing and may even provide opportunity to start the reflexive commentary on the experience.

The technicalities of interviewing

The purpose of the interview, alongside epistemological and methodological orientation will determine the nature of the interview. Brinkman and Kvale (2018) discuss the difference between the interviewer as a miner and a traveller. The miner, digging for precious metal (knowledge) that resides in the interviewee (an objectified reality) that is unearthed, without contamination by the interviewer (Brinkman & Kvale, 2018, p. 40), and the interviewer as a traveller who learns from the tales of others, co-constructs meaning and whose task is to tell that narrative to the research audience. The Miner metaphor is linked to a positivist, empiricist approach to data collection, one that seeks philosophical truths as much as mine for meaning in the unconscious (Brinkman & Kvale, 2018, p. 40), whilst the traveller metaphor is more linked to the social construction of reality (p. 41). Of note, no one approach is particularly right or wrong, the issue is which approach is taken to answer the research question and when that has been decided, to be consistent to that approach throughout the research process and in particular in report writing.

As an interviewer you are the research instrument. The extent to which you seek to remove yourself from data will be dependent on the assumed epistemological position. Either way, reflective notes written after episodes of data collection help to record the degree of objectivity that has been exercised or make transparent to an interpretivist the learning that has taken place from the interview.

As a health care professional, you enter the field with a distinct set of communication skills. Active listening, consciously attending to interactions, noticing responses, situation awareness, concentrating on mindful conversation, are all proficiencies that can be channeled into the research interview. However, the boundaries associated with the interviewer–interviewee relationship are dictated by the research purpose and ethical approval. Responding to a disclosure made in an interview that requires referral to another agency because what has been made known is either illegal or represents a danger to self or others, may be more skillfully handled because of professional training. The *sine qua non* is the interaction is determined by the research contract with the participant (made explicit in the information sheet and signed into the consent form): therapeutic intervention (bar an immediate crisis intervention and referral) is not a part of the process.

When entering the field, the primary role is that of interviewer. Like a graphic equalizer, the balance of other social and professional identities (e.g. self, teacher, nurse) may need to be suppressed to boost the energy and 'frequency band' of the researcher role. This is reflexively managed through hot, cool and analytical[4] field notes, but does require careful consideration and preparation prior to entering the field. There may come a point when the researcher role has to be abandoned

---

4   'Hot' refers to immediate responses to the field; 'cool' is with increasing distance from the field and 'analytical' describes reflection that is linked to methodological analytical procedure.

58   Julie Scholes

because too much distress has been invoked or to handle a disclosure (acts of omission and or commission). In the health, social care or education setting, the default is to then follow local governance procedure(s). The ethics committee will want to be assured you have a strategy in place to handle distress and disclosure. The funders will want to know the strategy you deploy will be effective and efficient.

Recording interview data

To protect anonymity and confidentiality data will need to be recorded using digital media A specialised microphone may prove to be a worthwhile investment to assure high-quality recordings for transcription. Charging, spare batteries and being able to operate the equipment might sound a patronising recommendation, but mistakes happen.

It is controversial to decide whether to take notes during an interview or whether the whole time should be spent attending to the interviewee. Note taking does have the benefit of keeping the interviewer focussed, drawing out items that might need further exploration at a later stage of the interview, highlight key theoretical insights and demonstrates to the interviewee you are taking them seriously. A hard-backed notebook and writing on one side of the book for data from the field with the left-hand page for analysis and reflective commentary (using different coloured pens to indicate whether it is hot, cold and or the stage of analytical review). When setting up the room take care to ensure you have the interview agenda in sight, the digital recorder placed for a good recording without being too confrontational and enough surface for all the paperwork.

Virtual interviewing

Although interviewing generates rich and insightful data, it is time consuming for the researcher but, more importantly, for the participant. Increasingly, researchers are reporting that recruitment to studies is 'challenging' and latterly, in health care, a struggle. To improve recruitment and to minimise inconvenience might be achieved using virtual media. Some participants might be reticent to talk other than face to face with the researcher present, but this may be mitigated by the topic where social distance through virtual media or a telephone interview are preferred (Weller, 2019). Sometimes pragmatic decisions have to be made and distal interviewing by phone, internet, videotelephony (Skype/FaceTime), or email are required because interviewees are located in prohibitive locations, e.g. war zones, where there are high-risk environmental dangers, live in different time zones, or too distant to reach within budget and timescales (Meho, 2006). The rationale for the chosen media should be clearly stated and quite explicitly, the interview agenda/schedule designed appropriate to that media (Brinkman & Kvale, 2018). Researcher convenience and cost makes an inadequate argument. Enabling participation of those who might otherwise not have been able to contribute, or the media can serve to displace potential embarrassment, or where culturally, face-to-face interviews are problematic, make sounder justification. Box 3.2 sets out the challenges and benefits of email interviewing.

Qualitative methods   59

BOX 3.2 EMAIL INTERVIEWS

Benefits	Challenges
• Increases access to: individuals in hard to reach localities dispersed groups experts and elite • Enables anonymous replies (sensitive subjects where embarrassment might be an issue). • Allows people who have difficulty with verbal expression and people who communicate using computer assisted technologies to participate. • Enables reaching participants in different cultures and who communicate in languages other than the researcher (allows for e-translation). • Can ask one question at a time. • Can follow up and delve into the replies with a further question. • Follow-up questions to build the interview can be paced and carefully presented. • Can offer multiple questions and invite the participant to choose which one to answer. • Convenient for participant to respond when it suits them (asynchronous data collection). • Provides time to consider a response and opportunity for editing. • Reduces cost of transcribing (material already in electronic format).	• Limits participation to those who have access to the internet. • Accuracy of response rate (non-delivery). • Capturing participation (request deleted before reading). • Opt-in now more complicated because of General Data Protection Regulation (EU GDPR, 2018) that individuals have to agree to be part of electronic lists. • Recruitment through invitations posted on: blogs, Twitter feeds, web pages, Facebook, radio or newspaper reports. • Limited by the literacy of an individual. • Clarity of the question – whether it is one that can be understood. • Missing probes • Delayed reply • Impoverished/economic replies resulting in thin data • Lack of clarity in meaning • Risk in determining authentic voice of participant • Social attribution impacting on replies • Ability to follow up if participant makes a disclosure of gives evidence of distress

(ADAPTED FROM MEHO, 2006)

Video telephony and the telephone interview

Video telephony (Skype, FaceTime, Google Hangout) as a media through which to interview participants is growing in popularity. Commercial video conferencing facilities are also used as part of the digital communication technologies. Telephone interviews raise similar issues but without the visual image. Convenience, accessibility and the use of a media that is familiar to many who communicate using the internet are dependent on good broad band width, a sufficient mobile data package, contemporary equipment that can upload the latest versions of the products, a working microphone and camera (Weller, 2019). The technology in use needs to be assessed to ensure no breach in confidentiality, intrusion or eavesdropping can occur (Cheng, 2019) and recording the interviews using apps that are embedded into the software requires careful scrutiny to be sure they are not stored on the cloud, where personal data cannot be secured (Ko, 2019). Further, where video calls are being recorded, the participant should be made fully aware with signed permission to proceed obtained prior to the recording. It may be that permission for verbal recording is granted and this can be achieved by placing a digital voice recorder beside the computer or phone and only using visual technologies as the medium to facilitate the interview.

Video telephony enables the building of rapport with participants, picking up on nonverbal cues, and with experience, can be as effective as face to face interviews. Probing and follow-up questions are as free flowing but care needs to be taken in not talking over the participant if they are any signal delays. They are particularly useful for participants who might fatigue easily (the interview can be broken down to smaller chunks and with consent of the participant, built over a number of days) and convenient for individuals who experience significant mobility issues or sensory challenges. The approach is useful to include participants who might not otherwise be able to contribute to the research because of time, distance or vulnerability (Weller, 2019). It provides participants with the ultimate power to discontinue an interview (hanging up), can accommodate last minute requirements to reschedule or create opportunity to speak with participants who spontaneously have something they wish to add or clarify from a previous interview. However, this can also be the Achilles heel with scheduled interviews forgotten or being superseded by other priorities. To cover this, it is important to determine with the participant as part of the consent process, how many times you can reschedule and send reminders without this becoming onerous.

Handling disclosures or distress will require practice to enhance remote assurance and crisis intervention strategies. The extent of that training will be linked to the sensitivities of the subject under discussion. As has been previously illustrated, you cannot be sure what sensitivities can be raised for another person by asking what may seem an innocuous question. However, attentive listening, noticing and generating distal empathy with participants will help to alert the interviewer to any discomfort. Determining when the interview should be discontinued, deferred or cancelled is an experiential matter but one where prior thought has been given to the boundaries of what is research data and what is personal. Once again, the wisdom of a health care professional can help to support these types of decision, but care needs to be taken not to assume a therapeutic role within the interaction that was established and consented to be for research purposes (Targum, 2011).

Qualitative methods **61**

Potential for problems with the technology require there to be an alternative mode of communication and it is wise to always have another contact number or email address provided by the participant in case of equipment failure (Meho, 2016).

In summary, video telephony can be an extremely effective means of conducting interviews. On occasion it might be a preferred option for participants who chose to remain in their personal space and communicate to a distal researcher (Brinkman & Kvale, 2018). It is a useful tool to balance the power between the researcher and researched where there is matched access to the relevant technologies, confidence and competence to use the equipment. This is not necessarily a generational issue, but it could be one related to finance and privilege. The medium is useful in longitudinal studies (Weller, 2019), for follow-up questions or for reaching individuals outside the original sample (for example in theoretical sampling). However, it is also a useful standalone interviewing tool and one that might be preferred to the telephone.

Focus groups

Group interviewing should only be used when seeking the contribution of either a heterogenous or homogenous group of between six to ten people. An object, text, event or image gives the group a focus on which to start the discussion. The subject should be suitable for group discussion. Sometimes sensitive subjects are best discussed in group to modify the potential for embarrassment (Sherriff, Gugglberger, Hall, & Scholes, 2014). However, focus group interviews cannot be considered confidential or private, even if they are situated in ground rules generated by the group (Morgan, 1997). Further, there can be no guarantee that individual recordings might be made by individuals and distributed through social media at the point of interview. Ground rules can determine the basics of behaviour but cannot be enforced unless bound by professional responsibilities.

Recording can be challenging but helped by using a multi directional microphone. Video recording of the group will require considerable planning, location of camera and agreement of all the participants. As a rule of thumb, if individual attribution of a quote is required, or observation of interaction between the group, carefully consider whether a focus group is the best media in which to capture these data.

Focus groups are exceptionally useful for market research, sensitising the researcher's focus on what matters to the people in the field[5] and in generating research questions for interviews. They are also invaluable for verification of research findings.

Managing a group interview is like conducting an orchestra and careful attention needs to be paid to enabling the silent members of the group to speak and

---

5   This is quite distinct from Public Involvement in Research when groups are brought together to sensitise the researcher to conduct in the field and issues that are most relevant to them. Focus groups collect data and require information sheets and consent. PPI involvement generates ontological practice but does not provide research data.

62 Julie Scholes

quietening dominant voices in the group. Capturing and collating the feedback in the group can be done using a flip chart which has the additional benefit as a device to demonstrate what data are being collected and getting immediate feedback that what has been captured has been accurately recorded and understood.

Practicalities include ensuring the room is appropriate and in a suitable location, that suitable furniture is laid out according to the requirements of the meeting. Allocating sufficient time to conduct the meeting but before it starts building the ground rules with participants. Providing refreshment and breaks may be necessary of the meeting is over an extended periods and breaks can be useful to de-escalate debates that get impassioned.

Practice is essential and Janesick (2016) offers some excellent exercises to build skills and capabilities in conducting a focus group. It is good practice to have a colleague who can facilitate the management of distress should it arise, take notes and generally offer assistance throughout the focus group meeting but also in the debriefing and cooling out procedures at the close of the interview.

Focus groups should not be used because of researcher convenience or as measures to reach targeted sample sizes. There should be adequate rationale in support of a focus group that privileges the participants and enables the exploration of a subject that captures common as well as idiosyncratic opinion. For a fuller discussion on focus groups see Barbour (2018), Krueger and Casey (2014) and Stewart and Shamdasani (2015).

The practice of observation

Observation as a research method is the act of careful watching for systematic analytic purpose. It is a method used in positivist research: where observation requires detachment of the researcher from the subject under observation (be that viewing matter down a microscope or telescope, or by watching social activity through a one way mirror) whilst naturalistic observation requires the researcher to enter the natural surroundings of subjects and watch their spontaneous actions.

Gold (1959) defined four observational roles: covert and overt; participant and non-participant. In reality these are on a continuum, but the extreme practice of covert participation or covert non-participation raises significant ethical issues. Justified as seeking to understand behaviour that is not influenced by the presence of the researcher (the Hawthorn effect), modern day implementation of such roles is normally associated with legal of journalistic investigation (exposé). Covert observation of individual's internet activity, or participating in chat rooms using a false identity to gather *research data*, all raise significant ethical and moral issues.

Observation for health care research has to venerate the rights of the individual to privacy, autonomy and respect. Observatories that collate epidemiological data that are non-attributable to individuals provide intelligence to forecast, identify patterns, processes and health outcome (Hemmings & Wilkinson, 2003). Specific ethical review and permission have been granted to collate health care data (sometimes from patient records) to inform policy, direct innovation and regulation (Trenell, 2018). To distinguish the two: epidemiologists observe data, whilst naturalistic researchers observe people, their behaviour and events, in context (Spradley, 2016). As such, the naturalistic observer has to exercise a relational ethic that constantly attends to considering the participants first, safeguarding their rights, interests and sensitivities, protects their anonymity and confidentiality as far as possible, gives voice to the participants (Coffey, 2018) respect and honour their contribution and recognises the risk taken in allowing their lives to be observed. The methodology will shape the observation method and the extent to which co construction, verification and analytical exchange is designed into the study.

Access

Negotiating governance arrangements to ensure entry to the field is a complex and time-consuming process. The procedure for gaining entry will be dependent on the field of inquiry, but entering as a participant observer will raise anxieties and concerns. Rather than assuming there will be no problems, assume there will be and work actively to head off reasons to deny access by gaining the participation of the people in the field to determine what would work for them and how. This can be translated into an observation protocol that can be invoked after it has gained the approval of the ethics committee and relevant stakeholders. The act of co-constructing the observation protocol demonstrates the ontological practice of the observer alongside the epistemological intentions and purpose of the research. This helps to assure participants because they are aware of what will happen, when and for what purpose. There is nothing covert, no intention to pry, interfere, meddle simply to learn from watching. The degree of participation assumed by the observer will also need to be agreed upon prior to entering the field. See Box 3.3 for an example story from the field.

BOX 3.3 EXAMPLE: TALES FROM THE FIELD

One of the first participant observation roles in an intensive care unit (ICU) was undertaken in a Nursing Development Unit (NDU). I wanted to watch practising ICU nurses and learn why patients in the care of some of those nurses appeared to be more comfortable, stable and settled. Prior to my gaining access to the field, management had commissioned a research group who examined employee activity. The aim was to determine how much of the activity undertaken by the nurses could be deployed to health care assistants or ward receptionists. The researchers were psychologists and social scientists who undertook an overt non-participant observer role, every five minutes recording activity against an observational check list from the vantage point of the nurses' station. One of those activities was listed as 'behind the curtains'. The nurses recognised quickly, that if they pulled the curtains, they were not being observed. The results of the study were significantly compromised, because what went on behind the curtains and delivered by qualified ICU nurses was where all the specialist expertise was practised.

Entering the field as a researcher who had been ICU nurse and was now a nurse lecturer, I was sensitised to the possibility that 'behind the curtains' was where I was most likely to observe the minutiae of practice that made a difference to patients (and their relatives, because the nurses pulled the curtains to avoid the 'prying eye' of the employment researchers, particularly in times of their distress). Recognising that my ICU skills were at best rusty (after two years at University undertaking postgraduate studies and four years lecturing), I asked the ICU team if I might assume the role of a student nurse working beside the qualified nurses. In this way, I could ask naïve questions of their practice,[6] serve some partial useful purpose as a pair of hands to help with turning, lifting and acting as a runner to fetch equipment, but also be beside the patient to witness the care they were given. This privilege was agreed because I was an ICU nurse by background. This is where I had the great honour to observe the therapeutic use of self put into practice by the ICU nurses alongside therapeutic absence (allowing the patient to rest and stabilise without intervention but with active and attentive observation of the patient's physiological parameters and nonverbal cues). The employment researchers had conceptualised this phenomenon as 'sitting: non-clinical activity').

Conduct in the field

The participant observer role in the health care setting raises significant issues. One key objection is the time an observed participant will have to consent to participate in the research. In busy health care setting not all people in the field will have had opportunity to read the information sheet and consent. Strategies to manage this include: to advertise widely by poster that the research is taking place, attend a range of multi professional and management meetings to advise people of the research, or attempt to limit the field (curtain off zones, but this might well compromise the naturalistic setting) and not record data relating to non-consenting persons in the field. In busy health care settings, minimising any disruption to normal practice and flow of patient care is not only wise, but pivotal to gaining access to the field.

When observing as a health care professional, one can witness incidents or practises that place an individual at risk.[7] In this event the researcher has to

6　This was made possible because a spate of full-time study and then assuming a lecturer role rendered me as an 'academic' and as consequence 'clinically clueless'.

7　The classic example is witnessing a cardiac arrest. The health care professional should take all necessary actions within their sphere of competence and the first of these will be to press emergency alarms and or immediately call for back up (if competent in Basic Life Support Skills, carry these out until help arrives). Not all incidents can be as dramatic or extreme, the most difficult to handle are where and when the circumstance is subtle. Seeking the counsel of the participants in the field is the better solution because their practice is current and they can guide action as they are aware of all clinical protocols.

Qualitative methods   65

abandon their researcher role and assume the professional code of conduct and comply with clinical governance arrangements. All this should have been made explicit in the participant information sheet and actions to be taken made clear in the co-constructed and verified observation protocol. Therefore, no action taken by the researcher should come as a surprise (See Archbold, 1986).

If the intention of the researcher is to be covert and making known the purpose and intentions of the research would affect behaviour and compromise the 'truth' of what is being observed, the question should be: is this research or an investigation?

Once in the field, building rapport, addressing researcher reactivity (on entering and leaving the field), becoming comfortable in the participant observer role, positioning, note taking, maintaining observational focus need to be consciously addressed through reflective field notes after each day in the field. Field notes can determine if the observer has gone native (Gold, 1959) i.e. they no longer see what there is to be researched rather participate in the social world without research purpose. This is easy to spot because the notes of the day will be brief and lack analytical insight. To address this, leave the field and undertake analysis of the data collected thus far to help regain focus. For conduct in the field, see Coffey (2018); Robson and McCarten (2016); Spradley (2016); Taylor, Bogdan, and DeVault (2016); and Burgess (2003), and for seminal texts on qualitative field work, see Schatzman and Strauss (1973), Geertz (1988), Lofland and Lofland (1995), and Sandelowski (2002).

If the researcher is seeking to undertake observation of professional practice, particularly in acute or critical care settings or situations, the most likely way to gain access to these situations is by reconstructing the field through high-fidelity simulation settings. Ontological deviations of the approach include constructing a defined time line for the observation and circumscribed the events that were to take place within the simulation laboratory on that time line. Therefore, the behaviour, decisions and actions are in response to an artificial scenario, devoid of other naturalistic influence and conditions. Simulation does provide proxy for the real-world situation and ever sophisticated technologies and virtual reality can provide a medium to gain critical understanding by 'being there' (Geertz, 1988, p. 1) albeit in a virtual capacity (see Box 3.4). However, access to the equipment and laboratories might require careful negotiation, working out of office hours and this might impact on recruitment. Provision for this should be costed in any research proposal.

BOX 3.4 EXAMPLE: THE SIMULATION LABORATORY AS PROXY FOR THE NATURAL SETTING

Locating the 'field' (Schatzman and Strauss, 1973) as the simulation laboratory was a pragmatic decision to avert the complex ethical challenges of being in clinical practice with the explicit purpose of awaiting clinical deterioration. It avoided photo elicitation of extremely unwell patients or non-consenting healthcare professionals who came to their aid. Although not ideal in terms of capturing naturally occurring events, it did provide a pragmatic solution to

> observing and gaining understanding of a phenomenon that is known to be problematic (NICE, 2007).
>
> Observing performance in a simulation laboratory is not without ethical concerns but they are more contained. For example, the researcher can offer immediate reflective review of the participant's performance and a separate debrief of their experience. Participants can learn from their error, without that error doing harm. Remedial training (lectures and additional simulations), to enhance performance and understating of clinical deterioration were prepared for those who requested it. Therefore, the research could serve as an educative opportunity, one that could empower the participants (Keller et al, 2008) and this in part, served to justify the use of the participant's time.

A postmodern approach to observation is to allow for the participant to review their own performance and provide an explanatory account of their actions (rather than the researcher determine what was happening and why) (Scholes, 1998). Video (and virtual reality) provides an excellent medium to enable this review. The researcher can sit beside the participant and learn what they know and how that knowledge informs their actions. Capturing multiple constructions of the simulation experience framed by all those involved provides nuanced and multi-layered insight into practice that might otherwise be off limits to a researcher. Video is more likely to be approved in simulation settings. However, secondary analysis of documentary footage might be a useful source; if necessary, permissions, copy right and access to original footage can be obtained. For the use of still visual images and film, see Banks (2018), and for visual ethnography, see Pink (2013).

Documents

When in the field, collecting documents, with necessary permission, is an important and helpful strategy to help contextualise and inform data analysis. Documents pertaining to the field can also be accessed online, but if these are available through an organisation's intranet, ensure you have consent to directly quote from them (always date and page reference as appropriate). Take care to distinguish between public and private records and ensure retrieval is compliant with the data protection act.

Documents as data may be used as additional supportive evidence or to provide balance where difference of opinion is revealed in the data. Documents can be a useful resource to help sensitise the researcher into the field but also understand different perspectives of various stakeholders that shape any particular context. For a fuller discussion on retrieving documents and documentary analysis see Robson and McCartan (2016, pp. 349–359) and Bowen (2016).

BOX 3.5 EXAMPLE: THE PRACTICE OF COLLABORATION – FINDING A PLACE FOR QUALITATIVE METHODS TO EMPOWER THE VOICE OF PEOPLE FOR WHOM THE RESEARCH IS BOTH FOR AND ABOUT

Working with colleagues in the Brighton Centre for Regenerative Medicine and Devices, we built a strand of activity called 'Sensitive Science' linking bench scientists with clinicians and patients to facilitate research (Scholes & Santin, 2017). Alongside helping scientists construct their lay reviews, pathway to impact statements, and facilitating public engagement. This includes discussion about what is considered morally acceptable, feasible and ethical alongside engaging the patients and their families about the acceptability of the science that is being proposed. In the past, beneficiaries of such an approach were considered to be the persons for whom the treatment was being developed. This model was generated from a knowledge exchange conference of key stakeholders including clinicians, bench scientists and the public and the emergent value set is sustained by continuing participation in our bid writing, reviewing, delivery of research, co-production of research and dissemination. The conference and the subsequent activities have clarified that all who participate in such an enterprise are beneficiaries. Therefore, at each point there is a tripartite meeting of clinicians, researchers and the patient and public.[8] Examples include the following:

The New Immortals: an art exhibition (2016) (https://www.phoenix brighton.org/events/the-new-immortals/) whereby the bench and social scientists and artists became one of the installations and created a space in a public art gallery in which they could meet and discuss with the public their work in the field of regenerative medicine.

Telematics[9] translations: interactive virtual art installation for health literacy on arthritis. The proposal involved the generation of a virtual art installation so the public could engage directly with the interior of a joint space that is damaged by arthritis and through interactive play show how regenerative medicine can contribute to arthritis treatments. The primary focus is to enable the public, patients, clinicians and scientists to consider, together, the implications of these treatments by raising their social and ethical imaginations and then to debate the wider societal implications of these treatments to improve the quality of life for people with arthritis. Drawing on techniques developed

---

8   The literature reports PPI occurring primarily as a bipartite relationship (Brett, Staniszewska, Mockford et al., 2014).

9   The telematics methods (Sermon & Gould, 2015) creates a virtual space in which people can become part of an educational video performance. Participants enter a 3x4 meter space, designed to simulate a joint damaged by arthritis and the performance is in demonstrating how the treatments work. Thus the audience become participants in the installation and through virtual means are projected onto a screen. It appears to the participant they are in the joint. The process of participation is intended to stimulate awareness and trigger deeper thinking about arthritis and how it can be managed.

from creative performance analysis and learning through simulation, the multi-disciplinary team proposed to implement this innovative ethnographic approach that places emphasis on co production, a relational ethic and built around a collective experience.

Diagnosing early stage Parkinson's and Alzheimer's diseases. The detection of early stage disease raises ethical issues and public sensitivities, particularly in the absence of efficacious cures. The social science team undertook interviews and focus groups with members of the public to explore how to guard against stigmatization and exclusion and to identify with people what mattered most to them.

Conclusion

Qualitative methods provide insight into the experience, feelings, perspectives and understandings of participants. It is rare outside research for an academic award to find research based on a single data collection method. The use of method should be consistent with the research question and epistemology and methodology will nuance the approach. A method should privilege the participants' contribution rather than the researcher's convenience. However, the method will need to convince a funder of the merits of the research design and if that is value for money. Qualitative methods are time consuming and will seek to recruit smaller numbers of participants and therefore sampling will need to take into account the rationale for who has been chosen as representative of a wider group. Analysed qualitative data can be shared with groups (focus groups or consensus conference) to engage wider participation.

Successful deployment of qualitative methods requires solid preparation, rehearsal, review and reflexive evaluation. The researcher is the instrument of data collection and therefore self as instrument needs careful attention to maintain poise, exercise high levels of attention, practice a relational ethic and be deeply considerate to those who agree to participate in the research. Working with people in the context you wish to research to identify how researcher conduct can be sensitive and minimise disruption and engaging patient and public involvement throughout the application of these methods is key. Putting into practice all the practical and theoretical components of any qualitative method is complex and can be challenging. Ensuring collegiate advice, wise counsel and debriefing after being in the field can help to dissipate the nerves, but nervous anticipation of entering the field is to be expected.

Qualitative methods provide rich data that serve to raise awareness and increase understanding of the participant's world. It is critical to ensure the voice of the participant is heard. That may mean building new alliances with colleagues from other disciplines and working in fields that might otherwise not have been considered (see Box 3.5). Just as the medium by which qualitative data collection has evolved, so too must the field researcher.

References

Archbold, P. (1986) 'Ethical Issues in Qualitative Research', p155–164 in Chenitz, W.C. and Swanson, J. M. (eds). From *Practice to Grounded Theory: Qualitative Research in Nursing Menlo Park*. CA: Addison-Wesley.

Banks, M. (2018) *Using Visual Data in Qualitative Research*. London: SAGE.

Barbour, R. (2018) *Doing Focus Groups* (2nd ed.). London: SAGE.

Bowen, G.A. (2016) 'An introduction to document analysis'. [Online at Research Methodology in Education] Available at https://lled500.trubox.ca/2016/244

Brett, J., Staniszewska, S., Mockford, C., Herron-Marx, S., Hughes, J., Tysall, C. and Suleman, R. (2014) 'Mapping the impact of patient and public involvement on health and social care research: a systematic review'. *Health Expectations*, 17(5): 637–650.

Brinkman, S. and Kvale, S. (2018) *Doing interviews* (2nd ed.). In U. Flick (Series ed.), *The SAGE qualitative research kit* (2nd ed.). London: SAGE.

Burgess, R. (2003) *Field research: A sourcebook and field manual*. Abingdon on Thames:Routledge.

Cheng, R. (2019) 'Apple fixes its FaceTime bug'. [Online; Accessed 4 February 2019] Available at www.cnet.com/news/apple-says-it-fixed-the-facetime-eavesdropping-bug-software-update-coming/

Coffey, A. (2018) *Doing ethnography* (2nd ed.). In U. Flick (Series ed.), *The SAGE qualitative research kit* (2nd ed.). London: SAGE.

EU GDPR.org (2018) 'The EU General Data Protection Regulation (GDPR) is the most important change in data privacy regulation in 20 years'. Available at https://eugdpr.org

Flick, U. (2018) *Designing qualitative Research* (2nd ed.). London: SAGE.

Geertz, C. (1973) *The interpretation of cultures*. New York: Basic Books.

Gold, R. (1959) 'Roles in sociological field observation'. Social Forces, 36, 217–213.

Hemmings, J. and Wilkinson, J. (2003) 'What is a public health observatory?' *Journal of Epidemiology and Community Health*, 57(5). http://dx.doi.org/10.1136/jech.57.5.324

Herbert, J. and Rubin, I. (2013) *Qualitative interviewing: The art of hearing data*. London: SAGE.

Janesick, V. (2016) *"Stretching" exercises for qualitative researchers* (4th ed.). Thousand Oaks: SAGE.

Keller, C., Fleury, J., Adriana Perez, A., Barbara Ainsworth, B. and Vaughan, L. (2008) 'Using Visual Methods to Uncover Context', in *Qualitative Health Research*, 18(3): 428–436.

Ko, E. (2019) '5 safety concerns with cloud data storage, answered viewed systems and software' [Accessed 4 February 2019] Available at https://systemsandsoftware.com/5-safety-concerns-with-cloud-data-storage-answered/

Krueger, R. and Casey, M. (2014) *Focus groups: A practical guide for applied research*. Thousand Oaks: SAGE.

Kvale, S. (1996) *InterViews: An introduction to qualitative research interviewing*. Thousand Oaks, CA: SAGE.

Lofland, J. and Lofland, L. (1995) *Analysing social settings: A guide to qualitative observation and analysis*. Belmont, CA: Wadsworth.

Meho, L. (2006) 'E-mail interviewing in qualitative research: A methodological discussion'. *Journal of the American Society for Information Science and Technology*, 57(10): 1284–1295. Avilable at https://staff.aub.edu.lb/~lmeho/meho-email-interviewing.pdf

Morgan, D. (1997) *Focus groups as qualitative research*(2nd ed.). London: SAGE.

Nandagiri, R. (2017) 'Why feminism: Some notes from the 'field' on doing feminist research'. [Online at London School of Economics and Politics; Accessed 6 February 2019] Available at http://blogs.lse.ac.uk/gender/2017/10/12/why-feminism-some-notes-from-the-field-on-doing-feminist-research/

National Institute for Clinical Effectiveness (NICE) (2007) 'Acutely ill adults in hospital: recognising and responding to deterioration'. [Online at NICE Pathways] Available at www.nice.org.uk/guidance/cg50

National Institute for Health Research (NIHR) (2019) 'Research passports'. [Online; Accessed 30 January 2019] Available at www.nihr.ac.uk/about-us/CCF/policy-and-sta ndards/research-passports.htm

Pink, S. (2013) *Doing visual ethnography*. London: SAGE.

Robson, C. and McCarten, K. (2016) *Real world research* (4th ed.). Chichester, UK: John Wiley and Sons.

Sandlowski, M. (2002) 'Re-embodying qualitative inquiry'. *Qualitative Health Research*, 12, 104–115.

Schatzman, L. and Strauss, A. (1973) *Field research strategies for natural sociology*. Englewood Cliffs, NJ: Prentice Hall.

Scholes, J. (1998) Therapeutic use of self: A component of advanced nursing practice. In G. Rolfe and P. Fulbrook (Eds.), *Advanced nursing practice*. Oxford: Butterworth Heinemann.

Scholes, J. (1995) *An exploration into the role transition of students converting from EN (general) to registered general nurses* (Unpublished doctoral dissertation). Sussex University, UK.

Scholes, J. and Freeman, M. (1994) 'The reflective dialogue and repertory grid: A research approach to identify the unique therapeutic contribution of nursing, midwifery or health visiting to the therapeutic milieu'. *Journal of Advanced Nursing*, 20(5): 885–893.

Scholes, J. and Santin, M. (2017) 'The beneficiaries model of patient and public engagement: The case for regenerative medicine'. Commentary on Research Translation Biomaterials Stakeholders in Europe,September 2017. Ingenio CSIC-UPV for the European Society of Biomaterials.

Sermon, P. and Gould, C. (2015) Occupy the screen | peoples screen. In S. Pop, T. Toft, N. Calvillo, and M. Wright (eds.), *What urban media art can do*. Stuttgart, Germany: AV edition GmbH, pp. 246–249.

Sherriff, N., Gugglberger, L., Hall, C., and Scholes, J. (2014) 'From start to finish: Practical and ethical considerations in the use of focus groups to evaluate sexual health service interventions for young people'. *Qualitative Psychology*, 1(2): 92–106.

Spradley, J. (2016) *Participant observation* (Reissued from 1980). Long Grove, IL: Waveland Press.

Stewart, D. (2016) 'Thinking beyond the bench' (Opening address). A Knowledge Exchange Conference, 1st March 2016.The Centre for Regenerative Medicine University of Brighton.

Stewart, D. and Shamdasani (2015) *Focus groups: Theory and practice* (Applied social research methods series, vol. 20) (3rd ed.). Thousand Oaks, CA: SAGE.

Taylor, S., Bogdan, R., and DeVault, M. (2016) *Introduction to qualitative research methods: A guidebook and resource* (4th ed.). Oxford: Wiley.

Targum, S. (2011) 'The distinction between clinical and research interviews'. *Innovations in Clinical Neuroscience*, 8(3): 40–44. Available at www.ncbi.nlm.nih.gov/pmc/articles/PMC3074196/

Tice, C. (2019) 'Make a living writing: Practical help for hungry writers' [Online, Accessed 1st February 2019]. Available at www.makealivingwriting.com/2-easy-tips-un-sucky-ema il-interviews/

Trenell, M. (2018) 'Healthcare in 2088 – how will research and innovation transform the NHS in the next 70 years?' [Online, NIHR Blog; Accessed 4th February 2019]. Available at www. nihr.ac.uk/blogs/healthcare-in-2088-how-will-research-and-innovation-transform-the-nh s-in-the-next-70-years/9012

Weller, S. (2019) 'The potentials and pitfalls of using Skype for qualitative (longitudinal) interviews' [Online, National Centre for Research Methods Working Paper 4/15; Accessed 1st February 2019]. Available at http://eprints.ncrm.ac.uk/3757/1/Susie%20Weller.pdf

UKCRC (2019) 'What is the UKCRC?' [Online, Accessed 29th January 2019]. Available at www.ukcrc.org/about-the-ukcrc/what-is-the-ukcrc/

4

THE PRACTICE OF GROUNDED THEORY

An interpretivist perspective

Julie Scholes

Introduction

Grounded theory is evolving. It had a beginning, there is a middle but as yet no end (Bryant, 2017). The antecedents to grounded theory, grounded theory's original authors, second generation scholars and practitioners have contributed to the generation of different schools of practice each with distinct philosophical assumption and method (Flick, 2018). To understand the diversity, one has to appreciate the history of grounded theory. Its history is steeped in politics and dominated by the discourses of the key protagonists and influenced by the era of their practice (Hallberg, 2009).

Learning how to practice grounded theory is experiential (Martin & Gynnild, 2011). *Doing* grounded theory teaches the researcher *about* grounded theory (Corbin, 2009). One necessarily has to front load the seminal texts, absorb these facts, be guided by the scaffold provided by the methodology and method, but understanding grounded theory is through doing and *trusting* the method. It is a personal researching experience and therefore becomes something more than the structural procedures that distinguish the approach. Its diversity/adaptability is both its strength but the target of critique.

These opening remarks make an implicit declaration of a social interactionist guided by the teachings of Leonard Schatzman (1991). A modest social scientist who worked with Glaser and Strauss as a co-researcher (Strauss, Schatzman, Bucher, Ehrlich, & Sabshin, 1963, 1964; Strauss & Schatzman, 1973), and teacher supervising PhD students and facilitating them with their analysis (Kools, McCarthy, Durham, & Robrecht, 1996). He did not participate in the political

72 Julie Scholes

debates, nor public discourse that marked out the first schism between the two founding authors (Gilgun, 2010).

Debates range from the intellectual 'ownership' of grounded theory,[1] when research can be considered a grounded theory, the acceptability of epistemological and ontological variants (Hallberg, 2009; Babchuk, 2011; Amsteus, 2014) whether grounded theory can evolve (Charmaz, 2006, Bowers & Schatzman, 2009) or if these variants simply reflect a school of qualitative methods (Glaser, 2008). The debate has led to labelling grounded theories (GT) with specific titles some omitting grounded theory in their title altogether, such as Glaserian GT and Straussian GT (Stern, 1995), Classic GT (Holton & Walsh, 2017), Dimensional Analysis (Schatzman, 1991), Constructivist GT (Charmaz, 2006), Situational Analysis (Clarke, 2005), and Grounded Theorizing (Bryant, 2017). It has been described as a methodology, a method, a technique, an approach (Bryant, 2017), a 'family of methods' (Bryant & Charmaz, 2007, p. 12) and a movement (Berterö, 2012). If you accept there can be variants of GT, then there are core procedures that unite the 'GT family' made distinct by the epistemological and ontological perspective of the researcher (Timonen, Foley, & Conlon, 2018). Therefore, when writing a grounded theory, it is essential to make explicit these philosophical positions and also to critically explain, elaborate and critique all the stages involved in building the theory (Amsteus, 2014).

A brief history of grounded theory

Glaser and Strauss had different scholastic roots: Strauss from the Chicago school of ethnography and symbolic interactionism; Glaser from Columbia University and a tradition of quantitative sociological method (multivariate analysis) to build middle range theories (LaRossa, 2005; Babchuk, 2011). Glaser subsequently argued that his analytical procedure (Classic Grounded Theory [CGT]) was systematic, drawing on the work of Merton, Lazarsfeld and others from Columbia University and that it included computational, mathematical procedure, to name but two techniques set out in *Discovery* and *Theoretical Sensitivity* (Glaser, 1992, p. 125). Strauss' work was influenced by the work of Goffman, Hughes, Blumer and Dewey with his approach to the field and analysis was steeped in the heritage of philosophical pragmatism. In *Discovery* they wrote about the fusion of these approaches.

In the 1960s they worked together at the University of California – San Francisco (UCSF) working with nurses and sociologists and built the doctoral programme that shaped the next generation of grounded theorists (Morse, 2009). Early in their tenure, they worked with Jeanne Quint (Benoliel), a nurse, and produced the first research conducted using the grounded theory method: *The awareness of dying* (1965). They wrote about the methodology in 1967 *The Discovery of Grounded Theory*. 'Discovery'

---

1   The politics of grounded theory maybe be broadcast through different contemporary media, but nevertheless, maintains the same fervency (see YouTube, tweets, web pages, Facebook pages, online colleges, journals, books – see for example, www.groun dedtheoryonline.com/who-we-are/ and www.groundedtheory.com).

was written to demonstrate rigor and robustness and complex processes to generate theory that could be considered a new approach to social research.[2] It was written at a time when paradigm tensions were at a peak and verifying theory, rather than generating theory was preeminent (Glaser & Strauss, 1967, p. 2). However, the actual process of data analysis remained elusive to most readers and established a thirst for more direction in the processes involved in handling data. As a consequence, two seminal texts were written, one by Glaser (1978), *Theoretical Sensitivity*, and one by Strauss in collaboration with his research student at UCSF and post-doctoral colleague, Julie Corbin, *Basics of Qualitative Research Analysis* (Strauss & Corbin, 1990). The latter book broke down into instructive parts, all the procedures associated with grounded theory, based on her working alongside Strauss and observing his method. It was the publication of this book that brought about an open critique and ruthless dissection of *Basics* by Glaser (1992), claiming the book undermined the constant comparative method and that grounded theory was his intellectual property: that Glaser was the true 'protagonist, propagator and proprietor'(Bryant, 2017, p. 91). Strauss allegedly was in Europe on a study tour whilst Glaser had written the bulk of *Discovery* in his absence. Glaser subsequently stated that common understanding was assumed, and alternative perspectives (or misunderstanding) only clarified in subsequent independent publications (Glaser, 1992). Therefore, Glaser argues that Strauss and Corbin started, and others have followed, to remodel the grounded theory method and reduce it to 'full conceptual description' or 'qualitative data analysis' if they stray from the original (his) approach (Glaser, 1992).

Glaser left academia and set up as an independent researcher and consultant, establishing Sociological Press (his own publishing house) in 1970 the Classic GT Institute in 1999 and CGT Website in 2008 and continues to provide seminars and workshops instructing research students in his method to ensure they do not 'force data' and obscure the 'emergence of theory'. In 2016 Grounded Theory On Line was established by 'Fellows', mentored by Glaser who in turn offer mentorship to students studying CGT.

Kathy Charmaz, a student of Glaser's introduced constructivist grounded theory (2006). Her approach uses greater reflexivity and an approach to co-constructing theory with participants (Charmaz, 2006) that distances itself from the 'objective' position (the authoritative voice of the researcher), sometimes referred to as the positivism evident in the original work and subsequent writings of Strauss and Corbin and Glaser.[3] Charmaz constructivist position embraces inductive,

2   When Glaser and Strauss wrote *Discovery* the legitimacy of social research based on interpretative method was under attack from the dominant discourse of positivism. Positivists wanted 'truth' and 'generalizability'. Discovery set out to communicate clearly the procedure of data collection and analysis to demonstrate robust, conceptual-analytical theory generation. The constant comparative method was at its heart (Glaser & Strauss, 1967, p. 1) and sets out a particular way of thinking about data (Morse, 2009).

3   Glaser's position on retaining objectivity with the data is an interesting one as Awareness of Dying was stimulated by recent losses both he and Glaser had experienced. However, Glaser has always espoused that the craft of the sociologist is to achieve analytical conceptualisation and that invariably subsumes the individual voice of participants. Glaser

74 Julie Scholes

comparative, emergent and open ended approach, alongside iterative logic and the dual emphasis on action and meaning described in *Discovery* but amplifies that research itself is a construction of multiple realities. Subsequently, Charmaz has written about symbolic interactionism and the impact this has on her approach (Charmaz, 2014). Latterly, she has written alongside Bryant (Bryant & Charmaz, 2007, 2011) who now claims three typologies of grounded theory: Straussarian, Glaserian and Charmazian and latterly Charmaz and Bryant (Bryant, 2017). Bryant's contribution has been in exploring the pragmatist heritage of grounded theory in his more recent work on grounded theorizing (Bryant, 2017, p. 328).

It is in the detail of the analytical procedure where divergence can be observed and alternative strategies deployed. Glaser argues, that in a randomised control trial no one would expect to see variability in procedure: so why tolerate it in GTM (Glaser, 2012)? His position is where authors avow variants, they describe an alternative qualitative method and therefore aren't Grounded Theory – they are other forms of qualitative analysis (Glaser, 1992). For analytical variance see Table 4.1. However, those who claim to use many of the techniques of GT and thereby label their approach: 'Grounded Theory' do so making explicit their epistemological and ontological rendering. Glaser rejects the notion of a given philosophical or theoretical perspective, put simply, those perspectives can be auditioned alongside any of the (CGT) coding families. Fostering a priori assumption (epistemological and ontological position), Glaser argues only serves to foreclose on what emerges from the data (Flick, 2018). One could argue that in making statements, Glaser himself is inadvertently declaring an empiricist position with a realist ontological bent (that the researcher as observer collects the facts from the field and through the inductive process of discovery, the theory emerges) (Amsteus, 2014). The researcher remains objective and then owns the data and represents the theory (Charmaz, 2014). Whilst schools where pragmatism and symbolic interactionism are acknowledged, co-construction in the field means participants and researcher work together to build a shared meaning and although the researcher makes explicit their reflexive position, the participants' voice takes precedence in representing the theory. This concept is based on a relativist epistemology and that theory is generated through abductive reasoning (inductive deductive cycles), meaning the researcher constructs an interpretive rendering of the participants' worlds. As such the theory is always partial, situated and subject to change (Charmaz, 2014). Glaser's perspective is to generate theory at a level of conceptual abstraction that has sufficient explanatory power that can explain a phenomenon irrespective of time and place. Indeed, *Awareness of Dying* has explanatory power and contemporary relevance more than 50 years after it was first published (Flick, 2018).

    also rejects the reflexive voice of the researcher despite advocating memo-ing to demonstrate the analytical decisions made during the research.

BOX 4.1 EXAMPLE: OBJECTIVISM – CONSTRUCTIVISM

These terms were used by Charmaz (2006) to distinguish her 're-modelled' constructivist grounded theory and to distinguish between co-construction and Glaser's position whereby theory is constructed by conceptualization and abstraction and based largely on an encyclopaedic knowledge of sociological theory. Glaser argues as theoretical construction begins this process transcends the contribution of any one participant, historical or situational context and therefore eliminates co-construction. Therefore, he gives priority to the researcher's analytic categories and voice and reflexivity as potential sources of data. Charmaz however, argues for multiple realities, assuming data are constructed through interaction in the messy world and views generalisations as partial, situated and located by time and context. Her aim is to give voice to the participants, recognising her own subjective position (managed reflexively throughout the process), with an aim of achieving an interpretive understanding of the situation under study. For a more detailed insight in to this debate, see Charmaz (2014, p. 235–241) for the constructivist position, and for a Classic Grounded Theorist perspective, see Simmons (2011, p. 19–27).

There is a strong apprenticeship tradition in grounded theory. The original authors supervised and supported the next generation of grounded theorists, who in themselves set about refining the paradigmatic, epistemological and ontological position and responses to critique and adaptations to enable action in contemporary society (Morse, 2009). Mentorship and a direct relationship with the originator(s) is advocated by Classic adherents (Martin & Gynnild, 2011), who suggest that people not associated with the original author(s) are responsible for the 'workarounds and extensions that have muddied the execution of the method' (Ibid., p. 5). Peer mentoring through networks is advocated to generate 'competent performers of *the* method' (my emphasis) indicating that Glaser persists in his quest through the website and Grounded Theory Institute, to perpetuate the notion that there is only one grounded theory: classic grounded theory, and developments are layers of maturation in that method. 'Minus mentorship' refers to persons who have not had direct contact with Glaser or his associates and suggests that misunderstandings are reproduced evidencing methodological inconsistencies.[4]

The key techniques of a grounded theory include the following features:

---

4   I declare myself as a 'minus mentor' author – whose contact with Glaser was via one skype seminar and with various interactions with a Classic GT Mentor but outside any formal Classic GT training programme. Interactions with Classic GT contributors has been through the Grounded Theory Special Interest Group at the University of Brighton where we have studied, critiqued, respected difference and embraced all generations and developments of the grounded theory method.

76 Julie Scholes

- When and what literature are reviewed to establish the research question
- Data analysis drives data collection
- The constant comparative method
- Coding and categorization (although different variants have different terms; see Table 4.1) driven by the data rather than pre-existing hypotheses/ theories
- Examining and making explicit the relationship between the categories
- Theoretical sampling
- Theoretical sensitivity
- Theoretical sufficiency/saturation
- Theoretical sorting
- Theoretical comparison (including auditioning theory)
- Iterative cycles of induction and deductive reasoning
- Conceptual abstraction
- Conceptual integration
- Memo-ing
- Relational ethic
- All is data
- Raison d'etre: to build theory
- Evaluative criteria: fit, grasp, workability, modifiability

The analytical process: the constant comparative method

The *sine quo non* of grounded theory method is the constant comparative method [CCM] (Hallberg, 2009): whereby data are compared within partici-pant data, across participants and against ever increasing circumstance or chan-ging conditions (e.g. time, stakeholder position, incidents, etc.).[5] The purpose is to see patterns within the data – and label those patterns (initially inductive codes but later using or borrowing codes from theories to label chunks of data) When codes are merged, they are known as categories. As codes and categories emerge, CCM continues to compare across the properties and dimensions of each category and as theoretical construction progresses, CCM involves com-parison with extant literature. Although the different elements of the GT ana-lytical method have been presented as discrete entities, they are iterative and interdependent.

Theoretical sampling

Theoretical sampling is a procedure whereby the researcher actively seeks data that can inform the constant comparative method. It differs from purposive sampling because by its nature, data are sought to confirm, refute or saturate categories that

5   Although Glaser would argue that through conceptualisation the coding and categor-isation of patterns is devoid of time, place and person (Glaser, 2002).

TABLE 4.1 Analytical variance

Glaser and Strauss, Discovery, 1967	Strauss and Corbin, Basics, 1990, 1998	Charmaz, Constructing, 2006	Schatzman, Dimensional, 1991	Classic, 1978 – to date
Coding technique/terms				

Codes
Concepts
Categories
	Open Coding
	Axial Coding
	Selective Coding
		Initial coding
		• Line by Line
		• Incident to incident
		• In Vivo
		  Focussed Coding
		• Axial coding
		• Theoretical coding
			Designation
			Perspectives
			• Naming data bits
			• organising
			  Dimension
			Properties
			Integration
				18. coding families
				1. Causes
				2. Contexts
				3. conditions.
				4. Consequences
				5. Co-variances
				6. Degree
				7. Dimension
				8. Interactive
				9. Theoretical
				10. Type coding
				11. Identity-self
				12. Means-goals
				13. Cultural
				14. Consensus
				15. Process
				16. Unit
				17. Cutting point
				18. Strategy
				Added in1998
				1. Paired opposite
				2. Representation
				3. Scale
				4. Random walk
				5. Structural functional
				6. Unit identity

Glaser and Strauss, Discovery, 1967	Strauss and Corbin, Basics, 1990, 1998	Charmaz, Constructing, 2006	Schatzman, Dimensional, 1991	Classic, 1978 – to date
Categories derived by				
Redesigning Reintegrating theoretical notions reduction	Linking action and interaction Inductive-deductive cycles	Emerging analysis through conceptualisation	Integration and linking through abductive reasoning	Conceptualisation and abstraction
Categories viewed in relation to:				
Dimensions Conditions Consequences	Context Conditions Consequences	Interpretative Understanding may include causal conditions but contingent on contextual conditions (p. 120)	Context Condition Processes Consequences	Conceptualisations of: Situations Social worlds Social contexts
End point of constant comparative method: pre first writing of draft				
Substantive Theory	The conditional matrix with central organising phenomenon linking all categories	Analytic framework that links theoretical concepts	Explanatory Matrix with central or key perspective	Emergence of Substantive Theory

The practice of grounded theory   **79**

have been inductively derived through data analysis. Theoretical sampling might also occur to enable the researcher to learn more about a category, the links between categories and or the context and conditions that have consequences on the emerging theory (Strauss & Corbin, 1988, 1990). Participants are the source of data, but they are invited to participate because of what they might be able to contribute to the evolving theory rather than predetermined population criteria. The process is largely elusive and inconsistent (Glaser, 2002) but the researcher is continually directed by what emerges in the data. Data collection is driven by data analysis, the iterative process (Glaser & Strauss, 1967), but theoretical sampling is driven by the codes, and categories that emerge and is directed by the pursuit of analytic possibility (Charmaz, 2014).

So when does the researcher know when to theoretically sample? A practical guide is in noticing and attending to: 'the dog that doesn't bark' i.e. the idiosyncratic comment or insight that can sometimes help the researcher recognise the significance of more commonly occurring themes within the data. Therefore, the researcher may wish to theoretically sample for sources of data to determine the limits of idiosyncrasy within a category. However, theoretical sampling might well require a further submission or amendment to the ethics committee should you seek to interview or enter a new clinical field that was not cited in the original submission. Therefore, the researcher has to have sufficiently robust theoretical grounds to pursue further data collection.[6] It is a common error to engage in more field work rather than pay detailed attention to the analytical process (constant comparative method) especially in the early stages when coding may seem a struggle and analytical insight elusive. However, simply collecting more data rather than theoretical sampling may create further delays, feed analytical misfiring and importantly, waste the valuable time of volunteers who are willing to participate in the study. In summary, theoretical sampling is directed by the emerging theory and memo writing is an important technique to enable the researcher to see where more data are required and create an audit trail of decisions (Birks & Mills, 2015) to theoretically justify the submission of an amendment to the ethics committee. A practical tip is to ensure you have ethical approval to return to participants who have already volunteered data, to explore emerging theoretical ideas: thus theoretically sampling within the original cohort, but directed by theoretical emergence to ask a set of different abstracted questions. An alternative is to recruit people outside the NHS (for example at professional conferences or through special interest groups), but ensuring all the necessary governance procedures have been negotiated prior to any theoretically sampled field work (again you can pre-empt this possibility by designing in such a data source into the original ethics application). One final caution, excited by theoretical possibility be careful not to enter the field: 'take hit and run' (Rienharz, 1992) from your theoretical sample

---

6   The first recommendation would be to go back to the data collected and see if a further iteration of constant comparison across incidents, across participants, between categories provides insight or if indeed there needs to be a return to the field to theoretically sample for further sources of data.

Theoretical sensitivity

Theoretical sensitivity is about self-knowledge, knowledge of the field that emerges from the iteration between data analysis and data collection, the researcher's intellectual history, theoretical knowledge, and theoretical wisdom applied to the everyday (Birks & Mills, 2015). Primarily, theoretical sensitivity refers to the researcher's capacity to recognize analytic possibility within the data and this is usually associated with emersion in the field and data analysis.

Theoretical possibility also refers to a process whereby 'extant' theory is used, in conjunction with new data, to elaborate and *extend existing* theoretical constructions inductively derived from the data (Glaser, 1978). Theory can be 'auditioned' and used to elaborate, extend or develop concepts (Glaser, 1978) as scaffolding rather than an imposition that forces data analysis. Glaser (1978) advocates that existing grounded theories can be useful to consolidate other substantive theories to guard against the proliferation of 'small islands of knowledge' and contribute toward theoretical sensitisation.

Theoretical saturation/sufficiency

Theoretical saturation is achieved when no new categories can be identified from the data. Theoretical saturation is an ideal state and has been reframed to theoretical sufficiency to indicate when there is sufficient robust evidence to demonstrate fit and grasp and linkage between categories. A grounded theory is always provisional (Glaser & Strauss, 1967, p. 40) because the researcher remains alert to emergent perspectives, continuous comparison to cases of increasing distance to see how far the theory will fit or to audition the claim of generalisability (1967, p. 111). Aldiabat and Le Navenec (2018) argue that it is the substantive argument that demonstrates theoretical saturation rather than any text book definition (perhaps no more helpful than when the allegoric: 'category envelope falls off the wall' containing all the relevant codes merged into that category). Sufficiency is the preferred term to denote when the data is rich enough to evidence meaning, the connection between or process that links categories, when there is sufficient depth and breadth of data to have workability, fit and be recognisable and where (or when) no new interpretations can be suggested (Amsteus, 2014).[7]

---

7   Often made by supervisors provoking the new grounded theorist. The intention here is to establish confidence in the categories – especially when determining the core category, central organising phenomenon or key perspective. It is also a strategy to enable the novice researcher to start to defend their theory –or to interrogate their data for alternative theoretical rendering.

Memo writing

The use of memos is critical in grounded theory. They are the system by which a grounded theorist makes evident their decision making and analytical thought process throughout the research process. Initially they can be grouped to distinguish or focus different types of thinking (through writing). Glaser advocates that memos can in fact be coded and categorized as a reflective oversight of the research process. The distinction between the constructivist and classic grounded theorist is in the reflective accounts that appear in the constructivist's analysis, whereas Glaser would assume these to be an audit trail of reasoning and conceptual abstraction. The different types of memo can initially be constructed as:

- Field work reflection (hot and cool, see Chapter Three)
- Sense making memo (clarifying your process, procedure and grasp of what is happening in the data)
- Analytical memo (starts with a question of the data and through comparative alinement of data raises a new question/perspective with which to view the data)
- Sampling memo (generating a clear rationale for theoretical sampling from the field or to rehearse theories for emergent fit)
- Preparatory memo (what conditions and context might impact upon data collected in the field, what sensitivities need to be recognized, what interactions need to be respected, any relational ethic that needs to be exercised)
- Theoretical memo (looking for patterns in the data that can inform theoretical explanation)
- Advanced memos (tracing the analytical procedure and conflating/integrating categories; relabelling, sorting and sifting; considering when theoretical sufficiency has been reached)
- Reflexive memo (making explicit researcher reactions, perspectives, interests and relationships with participants and representation of participants)
- Methodological memo (writing about grounded theory methodology, recording methodological activities and how they were implemented in the research, how the analytical procedure was enacted and how and when theoretical saturation/sufficiency was reached)

However, as the research progresses, the researcher may find different codes and categories to label their memos. See Heather Baid, Chapter Five.

Although memos might contain an emotional response to an experience in the field, supervision or critical self-review, their purpose is more than to journal or diarize the research experience: rather to condition a critical, deliberate act of abductive reasoning that can direct the next action (more data or more data analysis following a new line of reasoning). The act can enable a dialogue with the data and create opportunity for seeing all that is in the data through critical interrogation, an altered perspective or lens, and to illuminate analytical misfiring. They can

82   Julie Scholes

also be used to help focus theoretical sampling where gaps might appear of further data is required to address omissions or seek verification of emergent conceptualisations. Therefore, memos are critical to assuming a reflexive position but are a technique that is critical component of any grounded theory.

Memos can appear in the research report and should be clearly identified as a source. Examples of memos can appear in the appendix to help a reader understand the different types of memos and in an over view of the audit trail indicate how they relate to the sequencing of your data analysis and theoretical insight. Editing will be required as the process of memo writing can help to forge the authorial voice, but early drafts might require refinement before they make it to the public domain. Memos help the researcher to start writing from the outset. Memo writing forms a critical element but is not exclusive to the reflexive position.

The reflexive position

This is not simply an autobiographical account of how you came to the research topic and your experience along the research journey. It is a seasoned, analytical juxta position between self and data that sets out a clear audit trail of analytical decisions, the quest for openness and strategies assumed to achieve this, and a critical account of all stages of the research process. This is known as the reflexive position (Birks & Mills, 2015). The reflexive position is not a stream of consciousness, an act of confession, nor an intimate disclosure of your personal life but should indicate where circumstances should be taken into account (Charmaz, 2014, p. 241). Refining such statements and recognizing where they should appear is rehearsed through memos but evidenced through the sorting, labelling, categorization of memos and made explicit in the audit trail. In a report or thesis, the reflexive position can be located as a dialogue with the text in the form of footnotes. However, where the reflexive position is key to theoretical development (analytical insight) as an edited piece, labelled clearly as evidence to inform the systematic building of the substantive theory.

Openess is often considered to be the act of entering the research process without a priori hypothesis or pre-determined ideas. This can relate to assumptions from the literature and also personal values and ideas. Glaser (1978) is most clear that the researcher should remain both open and objective but, not empty headed. Charmaz introduced the idea amplifying the teachings more acknowledged in the Straussarian lineage (largely developed out of symbolic interactionism) that the researcher does not, nor can they, enter the field without any prior knowledge or personal bias. Indeed, the final chapter of *Discovery* does make mention of this (and if legend be true, this was chapter was written by Strauss, although the paragraph opens with '*Our* point'), and states: one should deliberately cultivate reflections on personal experience (Glaser, 1967, p. 252), . . . other people's experience . . . and insights from the literature (Glaser, 1967, p. 253).

Keeping an open mind needs active attention. Memos help the process of self-recognition alongside discussions with peers and supervisors. A useful strategy is to

The practice of grounded theory **83**

explore one's own personal bias and use this to interrogate the data. For example: If you were buying a property what might you notice? If you were the estate agent selling the property what would you notice? If you were offering a quote for removal fees by a removal firm what would you notice? If you were the lawyer undertaking conveyancing: what would you notice? This perspective searching is one strategy to notice any: 'ideation baggage to give up or correct' Glaser (1978, p. 44).

BOX 4.2 REFLEXIVE INTERROGATION

Hendley (2014) a midwife and passionate exerciser wanted to research the factors that influenced women's choice to exercise during pregnancy. She had to attend to her inherent belief that a) pregnancy was a welcome condition for all women, b) that physical change associated with pregnancy was marvelled and valued c) that exercise was viewed by pregnant women as a means of improving their labour and the wellbeing of the child. To help her handle her own values and beliefs she had to interrogate the data with questions such as: is their evidence within the interview data that pregnancy was not welcome? Was their any evidence in the data that indicated women grieved for the loss of their former figure? What if women exercised for their own pleasure and undertook exercise without consideration for the growing foetus?

Glaser argues that the way to maintain openness is to go conceptual – but also in the use of constant comparison. If something emerges here, can it be seen there? (Glaser uses the example from *Awareness* about dying in intensive care and dying on a cancer ward). Ethical approval now can limit quite severely the range of locations one can seek out data and being driven by theoretical sensitivity arising from the data to prompt theoretical sampling may be more limited than studies undertaken in the 1960s (Charmaz, 2014).

These ways of challenging the data can be set out in memos – some extended and labelled (and potentially sorted and relabelled at a later date). They can generate new labelling and coding frameworks / grids and should start with an analytical comment / question driving the collation of material to see what is in the data comparing across interviews, context, and indeed under different circumstances. The grids can end with either a theoretical memo or further analytical probing memo to take you to the next round of data collection (theoretical sampling) or data analysis. The end of each working day should always result in a Post-it note of sticker that directs your analytical activity/ field work for the following day. Where there is significant difference in direction make a reflective note of why you have diverted – either because of new insight, redirected reading, changed plans – or deep-down avoidance? All the time you are driving yourself toward theoretical reasoning that arises out of the data. This keeps you openminded but purposive and going conceptual is also important to allow for rising above the minutiae of detail to the process that is emerging through the analytical cycles. Writing memos is critical to enable the researcher to focus but also attend to the drive for conceptualisations.

Conceptualising and abstracting

Conceptualising and abstracting are done through abductive reasoning – involving inductive and deductive cycles. Laddering codes (and associated data) for comparison helps to focus induction and deduction. And produces evidence to illustrate the breadth, depth and scope of the category as well as links to other categories. This rigorous procedure can illuminate perspectives, entrenched ideas or analytical misfiring. Students mystified by the process of interpretation can often doubt the abductive process, fearing they have 'made up' an outcome. This soon becomes evident when there is insufficient evidence in support of the claims that are made and the reader finds gaps, senses inadequacy, or can impose an alternative explanation. Memo writing should illuminate these errors long before they become drafts for an external audience. However, submitting drafts and ideas for critical review from fellow grounded theorists can help to build confidence.

BOX 4.3 ORGANISING DATA

In generating new grids, guard against 'rearranging the deck chairs on the Titanic' (a very common issue) – whereby the student of grounded theory cannot move their thinking and just re order the content of any CCM grid often focusing on the concrete or literal rather than conceptualizing and abstracting meaning. To quote another instruction from all the authors of GT: 'all is data'. Ideas can be stimulated, for example, from listening to a debate on the radio on a topic that is quite distinct from the research but raises questions that can help you see new theoretical possibility in your data. The trick is in using these ideas as conceptual levers (Glaser, 2002) that help one grasp new insight and triggers further constant comparison. It may be that conceptual labels can be found searching terms online and auditioning their potential. This can and should be done with extreme caution and willingness to remain open. It is a useful strategy for lifting analytical block if treated as an invigorating, therapeutic and creative remediation, but should be time limited and a very tight audit trail maintained.

The literature review

It is a myth that grounded theorists enter the field without having first examined the literature. The argument needs to address why the topic is both timely and topical and why the methodology is appropriate (i.e. that little is known about the subject and what is being examined is a social process). The purpose is to set out the context and conditions into which you are locating the research with sufficient open mindedness to demonstrate that you are aware of what is already known and clear about what you are seeking to understand – without foreclosing on the likely theory to explain what emerges from the data. Kools et al. (1996) describe the review process as a 'conceptual entrée'.

The practice of grounded theory   **85**

In writing the initial review (research proposal), the researcher can stamp an authorial command by demonstrating an awareness of the key debates, issues, concerns and contested wisdoms in, and of, the field. This is quite different from embracing the arguments and evidence and then forcing that on your analytical thinking. However, you can audition theories and use them as conceptual levers to help with coding and categorization. *But,* always retain an open mind until you achieve saturation that you have arrive at an analytical insight that is fully connected, evidenced by examples and offers theoretical insight into the research question. Glaser (1978) has argued that you might alight upon the theory from day one of data collection analysis – but the trick is to keep going and retaining an open mind until no other theory can explain what is going on in your data (theoretical saturation).

Another key feature is to capture both seminal texts and recent research to demonstrate the depth and breadth of your grasp of the topic. This is important so that you can later demonstrate what is original in the work you have produced but also, to start the process of thinking for the reader about what needs to be discovered and how your research fills that gap. Writing a thesis is often done in stages with the literature review to position the research proposed research and potentially revisited at various stages of review (either made by research committees, or submissions to steering groups where the research is commissioned). What is important to note is the literature does need to be kept up to date and is constantly being revisited. The final edit of the review for the thesis will also transform to alert the reader much more explicitly to what the research will reveal because in a grounded theory it is not until the final write up that you know what your theory actually is and what literature needs to go where. Simply put, sections will often move, conceptualisations of the review reframed and the sense making process of the entire thesis edited together. It is a movable feast right up to the last iteration before sending to print and binding.

BOX 4.4 WHEN TO REVIEW THE LITERATURE

The initial literature review is unlikely to cover the sociological theory that emerges from the analytical procedure. For example, Trapani (2016) set out to examine factors influencing critical care nurses' decision making with regards referral to other colleagues. His theoretical explanation was dual agency. His initial research proposal and ethics application set out the literature on decision making but it was not until he had generated his explanatory matrix that he then started to review the literature on agency, moral agency, structure-agency integration and finally dual agency.

Likewise, Simmons (2019) set out to determine fathers' experiences following a premature birth. Her theoretical explanation of their experience: moratorial fathering explained how they endured sustained uncertainty in the transition to premature fatherhood. Her initial literature review examined parenting and fathers' experiences of having a premature baby on a Neonatal Intensive Care Unit and following discharge home but it was only after she had developed her substantive theory that she thoroughly explored the literature on uncertainty, situated fathering and identity and boundary ambiguity. In this way she prevented a priori

86 Julie Scholes

> assumption of the social process experienced by the fathers in her study but used the theoretical literature as a comparative source much later in the analytical process and in writing, to inform her discussion.

Therefore, a comprehensive review of the literature that approximates the substantive theory is delayed until data analysis drives that theoretical comparison. Also, there is considerable time dedicated to theoretical comparison with a number of theories auditioned to see if they have fit and grasp and if not, they are rejected. Preventing foreclosure is in keeping an open mind throughout and continuing to look for potential in the data that might not otherwise have been recognized.

Writing a grounded theory

Writing starts from the outset and should be encouraged from the earliest encounters with data and a recording of experiences in the field (or indeed the research process). Working with data and illuminating what has been learnt from the field, texts, experience needs to transpose into prose. At an early stage these are referred to as memos (Glaser & Strauss, 1967; Charmaz, 2014) but also field notes, reflective notes (Schatzman & Strauss, 1976). There is a difference in writing for analysis and writing for an audience (Charmaz, 2014).

> ### EDITING
>
> Some practical guidance when writing a grounded theory. There will be much editing. The editing can start from outset but in each iteration and stage of the research process, there will be revision. The final presentation is a result of many years hard work and that has to be reduced to a two-dimensional account of a four dimensional process. This can be extremely painful.

The following guidance relates to key chapters. In writing the methodology, do not provide a textbook account but use the literature to provide rationale for the actions/decisions that have been taken.

Write about the application of method to the context of your research, using examples from the field and (data) to illustrate the core techniques that you have used. By the end of the data analysis the reader should not be surprised by the substantive theory; i.e. the substantive theory demonstrates how all comes together as a process, provides explanation and has explanatory power. When introducing concepts be careful to provide evidence of them before you make conceptual headings, and when referring to a sociological concept ensure there is definition or explanation. Avoid colloquialism in the writing and focus on being analytical.[8]

8   This is different from using in vivo quotes or codes.

The practice of grounded theory   **87**

In writing the substantive theory determine if you are going to present literature as comparison against specific elements of your findings. Always remember to make explicit the choices made for the presentation of quotes: because they reflect the category or theme or because they reflect idiosyncratic difference. Do not be afraid to reflect how often this theme code, category appears. Be clear and communicate what your theory actually is. This takes repeated attempts.

Data are historic (and plural). Because data were given in a context and time that might differ from the reality of the participants world at the time of publication, and because the data has been interpreted presenting the findings in the past tense gives a gravitas and respect to the philosophical assumption that things change, processes are temporal, knowledge can only be partial and has been constructed (through rigorous analytical procedure) for the audience (Charmaz, 2014).

IMPACT

It might be that you hold back a quote that captures the essence of your theory as the final statement in your thesis. This is a quote that is powerful, memorable and has impact. Concluding with a participant's voice demonstrates how the espoused epistemological and ontological values have been put into practice. However, such a decision would require consistency with the variant of grounded theory that has been declared.

Writing the discussion

When writing the discussion, go conceptual. This is when you compare your substantive theory to formal theory. This is achieved by not going over the minutiae of codes and categories or, as is often the temptation to dissect back to the elements of the substantive theory. It might be that the discussion chapter starts with a summation of the substantive theory that is represented diagrammatically. Ensure that you start to allude to the formal theory within the substantive theory but take care to ensure this does not imply any forcing. There should be no surprises, but the gift is in enabling the reader to discover through your writing, the sociological process you have researched and theorised. Be careful not to introduce so many theories that it appears you are still auditioning theories in your discussion and or, have not yet reached theoretical sufficiency/saturation.

Writing the implications

Ensure there is evidence in your substantive theory for each implication (and not go beyond the boundaries of your thesis). Conceptualisation and abstraction continue, and new arenas for constant comparison will emerge after you have completed the thesis. This can be useful for post-doctoral work but be careful not to overstate your findings and extrapolate beyond the confines of what your theory discusses (Holliday, 2016).

Writing the limitations

It is often the case this section is written when tired or fighting the deadline for final submission. Researchers can find themselves writing a grand critique of grounded theory or even qualitative research per se: i.e. apologising for the sample size, the case context limiting generalisability etc. This weakens all the argument and rationale for decisions that should have been presented throughout the thesis. Therefore, it is recommended that you use grounded theory evaluative strategies about fit, grasp, workability, modifiability (Glaser, 1978, pp. 4–5; Holton & Walsh, 2017, Ch. 10) or usefulness, originality, credibility, resonance (Charmaz, 2014, pp. 337–338) and procedural precision. Therefore, the following issues can help to construct this section. Remember the reader has completed reading your thesis and does not want to be told they have wasted their time because it is entirely deficient with the limitations section reading like a public apology. However, this does not preclude a deeply theoretical and critical reflection on the following.

- Audit trail
- Memo-ing
- Reflexive position
- Data management
- Appropriate application of method to field – adaptations explained and justified
- Logical connections between concepts
- Discussion conceptual / theoretical explanation
- Theory evidenced in the data

Concluding remarks

Undertaking a grounded theory is a lengthy project (Flick, 2018). Learning how to do a grounded theory is experiential. When determining which variant of grounded theory you seek to follow, be consistent with that approach (following epistemological, ontological and theoretical maxims). It might be with experience and in different contexts allegiance to any one approach may shift (Timonen et al. 2018). However, be confident that you have adequate grasp of the methodology and methods and can position your theory with sufficient evidence from the data to lay claim to the approach being a grounded theory. Surround yourself with grounded theorists, engage in debate, seek critical feedback and review. Keep writing! Finally, and most importantly, trust the process.

References

Aldiabat, K.M. and Le Navenec, C. (2018) 'Data Saturation: The Mysterious Step in Grounded Theory Method'. *The Qualitative Report*, 23(1), 245–261. Retrieved from http s://nsuworks.nova.edu/tqr/vol23/iss1/18

Amsteus, M. (2014) 'The Validity of Divergent Grounded Theory Method'. *International Journal of Qualitative Methods*, 13(1), 71–87. Retrieved from https://doi.org/10.1177/160940691401300133

Babchuk, W. (2011) 'Grounded Theory as a "Family of Methods": A Genealogical Analysis to Guide Research'. *US-China Education Review*, A(3), 383–388.

Berterö, C. (2012) 'Grounded Theory Methodology—Has It Become a Movement?' *International Journal of Qualitative Studies Health and Well-being*, 7. doi:10.3402/qhw.v7i0.18571

Birks, M. and Mills, J. (2015) *Grounded Theory: A Practical Guide*. Los Angeles: SAGE.

Blumer, H. (2005) *Symbolic Interactionism: Perspective and Method*. (Originally published in 1986). Berkley, CA: University of California Press.

Bowers, B. and Schatzman, L. (2009) Dimensional Analysis. In Morse, J., Stern, P., Corbin, J., Bowers, B., Charmaz, K. and Clarke, A. (Eds.), *Developing Grounded Theory: The Second Generation*. Walnut Creek, CA: Left Coast Press, pp. 86–126.

Bryant, A. (2017) *Grounded Theory and Grounded Theorising Pragmatism in Research Practice*. New York: Oxford University Press.

Bryant, A. and Charmaz, K. (2007) Grounded Theory Research: Methods and Practices. In Bryant, A., Charmaz, K. (Eds.), *The SAGE Handbook of Grounded Theory*. London: SAGE, pp. 1–28.

Bryant, A. and Charmaz, K. (2011) Grounded Theory. In Williams, M. and Vogt, P. (Eds.), *The SAGE Handbook of Innovation in Social Research Methods*. London: SAGE.

Charmaz, K. (2006) *Constructing Grounded Theory*. Thousand Oaks, CA: SAGE.

Charmaz, K. (2014) *Constructing Grounded Theory* (2nd ed.).Thousand Oaks, CA: SAGE.

Clarke, A. (2005) *Situational Analysis: Grounded Theory After the Postmodern Turn*. Thousand Oaks, CA: SAGE.

Corbin, J. (2009) Taking an Analytic Journey. In Morse, J., Stern, P., Corbin, J., Bowers, B., Charmaz, K. and Clarke, A. (Eds.), *Developing Grounded Theory: The Second Generation*. Walnut Creek, CA: Left Coast Press, pp.35–54.

Denzin, N. and Lincoln, Y. (1994) Entering the Field of Qualitative Research. In Denzin, N. and Lincoln, Y. (Eds.), *Handbook of Qualitative Research*. Thousand Oaks, CA: SAGE, pp. 1–17.

Flick, U. (2018) *Doing Grounded Theory: The Sage Qualitative Research Kit*. London: SAGE.

Gilgun, J. (2010) 'An Oral History of Grounded Theory: Transcript of an Interview with Leonard Schatzman'. *Current Issues in Qualitative Research*, 1(10). Retrieved from www.scribd.com/doc/45707977/An-Oral-History-of-Grounded-Theory-Transcript-of-an-Interview-with-Leonard-Schatzman

Glaser, B. (2012) 'A Masterclass on Theoretical Sensitivity with Barney Glaser' [Skype Seminar] 3rd May 2012. The Grounded Theory Special Interest Group, University of Brighton, with Tom Andrews.

Glaser, B. (2008) 'Conceptualization: On Theory and Theorizing Using Grounded Theory'. *International Journal of Qualitative Methods*, 1, 23e38. Retrieved from https://doi.org/10.1177/160940690200100203

Glaser, B. (2007) Doing Formal Theory. In Bryant, A. and Charmaz, K. (Eds.), *The SAGE Handbook of Grounded Theory*. London: SAGE, pp. 97–113.

Glaser, B. (2002) 'Constructivist Grounded Theory?' *Forum Qual Sozialforschung/Forum Qual Social Res* 2002(3).

Glaser, B. (1978) *Theoretical Sensitivity*. Mill Valley, CA: Sociology Press.

Glaser, B. (1992) *Basics of Grounded Theory Analysis: Emergence vs Forcing*. Mill Valley, CA: Sociology Press.

Glaser, B. and Strauss, A. (1965) *Awareness of Dying*. New Brunswick, Canada: Aldine Transaction.

Glaser, B. and Strauss, A. (1967) *The Discovery of Grounded Theory: Strategies for Qualitative Research*. New Brunswick, Canada: Aldine Transaction.

Hallberg, L. (2009) 'The "Core Category" of Grounded Theory: Making Constant Comparisons'. *International Journal of Qualitative Studies on Health and Well-being*, 1(3), 141–148. Retrieved from https://doi.org/10.1080/17482620600858399

Hendley, J. (2014) *Women's choice to exercise during pregnancy*. Unpublished PhD, University of Brighton.

Holliday, A. (2016) *Doing and Writing Qualitative Research* (3rd ed.).London: SAGE.

Holton, J. and Walsh, I. (2017) *Classic Grounded Theory Applications With Qualitative and Quantitative Data*. London: SAGE.

Kools, S., McCarthy, M., Durham, R. and Robrecht, L. (1996) 'Dimensional Analysis: Broadening the Conception of Grounded Theory'. *Qualitative Health Research*, 6(3), 312–330.

LaRossa, R. (2005) 'Grounded Theory Methods and Qualitative Family Research'. *Journal of Marriage and Family*, 67(4), 837–857. Retrieved from https://doi.org/10.1111/j.1741-3737.2005.00179.x

Martin, V. and Gynnild, A. (2011) *Grounded Theory: The Philosophy, Method and Work of Barney Glaser*. Boca Raton, FL: BrownWalker Press.

Morse, J. (2009) Tussles, Tensions and Resolutions. In Morse, J., Stern, P., Corbin, J., Bowers, B., Charmaz, K. and Clarke, A. (Eds.), *Developing Grounded Theory: The Second Generation*. Walnut Creek, CA: Left Coast Press, pp. 13–23.

Reinharz, S. (1992) *Feminist Methods in Social Research*. Oxford: Oxford University Press.

Simmons, O. (2011) Why Classic Grounded Theory. In Martin, V. and Gynnild, A. (Eds.), *Grounded Theory: The Philosophy, Method and Work of Barney Glaser*. Boca Raton, FL: BrownWalker Press.

Simmons, S. (2019) *Moratorial Fathering: Enduring Sustained Uncertainty in the Transition to Premature Fatherhood* (Unpublished doctoral thesis). University of Brighton, UK.

Stern, P. (1995) Eroding Grounded Theory. In Morse, J. (Ed.), *Critical Issues in Qualitative Research Methods*. Thousand Oaks, CA: SAGE, pp. 212–223.

Schatzman, L. and Strauss, A. (1973) *Field research Strategies for a Natural Sociology*. Cambridge: Pearson.

Schatzman, L. (1991) Dimensional Analysis: Notes on an Alternative Approach to the Grounding of Theory in Qualitative Research. In Maines, D.R. (Ed.), *Social Organization and Social process*. New York: Walter de Gruyter.

Strauss, A. and Schatzman, L. (1973) *Field Research: Strategies for Natural Sociology*. Upper Saddle River, NJ: Prentice Hall.

Strauss, A., Schatzman, L., Bucher, R., Ehrlich, D. and Sabshin, M. (1963) The Hospital and Its Negotiated Order. In Freidson, E. (Ed.), *The Hospital in Modern Society*. New York: The Free Press, pp. 147–168.

Strauss, A., Schatzman, L., Bucher, R., Ehrlich, D. and Sabshin, M. (1964) *Psychiatric Ideologies and Institutions*. New York: Free Press of Glencoe.

Strauss, A. and Corbin, J. (1988) *Basics of Qualitative Research: Grounded Theory Procedures and Techniques*. Newbury Park, CA: SAGE.

Strauss, A. and Corbin, J. (1990) *Basics of Qualitative Research: Grounded Theory Procedures and Techniques* (2nd ed.). Newbury Park, CA: SAGE.

Timonen, V., Foley, G., and Conlon, C. (2018) 'Challenges When Using Grounded Theory: A Pragmatic Introduction to Doing GT Research'. *International Journal of Qualitative Methods*, 17(1). Retrieved from https://doi.org/10.1177/1609406918758086

Trapani, J., Scholes, J. and Cassar, M. (2016) 'Dual Agency in Critical Care Nursing: Balancing Responsibilities Towards Colleagues and Patients'. *Journal of Advanced Nursing*, 72 (10), 2468–2481. doi:10.1111/jan.13008

5

ENGAGING WITH GROUNDED THEORY RESEARCH AS A DOCTORAL STUDENT

Heather Baid

Developing a philosophical position

The research process begins with a hunch that new knowledge is needed to address a problem related to something unknown about a specific topic. A gap in the knowledge base, therefore, presents an opportunity for researchers to fill this void with innovative information developed from the research. The end outcome could describe, explain, generalise, correlate, show causation, predict, change, empower or deconstruct, depending on the type of question asked and how the researcher attempts to answer the question. However, postgraduate students on research-based programmes face challenges with the complexity of studying 'what' research is (including different types), alongside planning 'how' to conduct their research. My journey as a doctoral student began by designing the research while concurrently learning about various philosophical viewpoints of the research process. Acquiring a philosophical position became a central component of my ability to transition the research problem forward into suitable research questions to initiate the project design. See Figure 5.1 for an illustration of the steps involved during this introductory phase of the research process, as guided through increased awareness of my philosophical positioning.

Understanding my philosophy specifically came from reflecting on these two fundamental concepts, included as the middle steps in Figure 5.1:

- *Ontology* – nature of reality about what exists by asking what is there to know about the topic? Example ontological positions: realism and relativism.
- *Epistemology* – the type of knowledge acquired for what is sought to be known by asking how can I know about the topic? Example epistemological positions: positivism, interpretivism and constructivism.

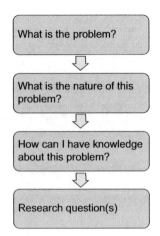

FIGURE 5.1 Initiating the research process from a philosophical positioning

Many novice researchers find these '-ology' and '-ism' terms daunting and difficult to grasp (O'Leary, 2017). I too found it strenuous to move beyond a superficial appreciation of their definitions into a sufficiently deep enough comprehension to confidently articulate my own ontological and epistemological position. At the beginning, I could not see a link between these abstract concepts and their practical application to the research design planning. Clarity on their usefulness came through multiple iterations of studying their meaning and the pragmatic action of 'having a go' with declaring my ontological and epistemological assumptions. Moving back and forth between learning about philosophy terminology and justifying my viewpoints led to further insights and eventually a richer understanding of how to both find and articulate a philosophical stance. See Table 5.1 for an overview of activities and practical examples I used to develop and express my own ontological and epistemological positioning for the PhD research project.

Choosing grounded theory

Once a research question or questions have been developed, the next phase of the research process involves identifying a suitable methodology to explain 'how' to undertake the research, along with methods for procedures on 'what' specifically will happen. The researcher may consider whether grounded theory research is an appropriate methodological choice for the design, although it can be difficult for postgraduate students to fully understand what grounded theory is (and equally, what it is not). In Chapter four, Julie Scholes highlights the experiential nature of learning grounded theory, best understood through 'doing' and 'trusting' in the process. However, the 'doing' can only occur once planning, approving and implementing the research. The novice researcher may

TABLE 5.1 Activities to develop ontological and epistemological positioning

Activities to help learn about research philosophy terms and concepts

Activities	Practical examples
Face-to-face teaching	Attend lectures, study days and workshops about research methodology and methods to formally learn the terminology and concepts
Reading scholarly and online publications	Read textbooks, journal articles and websites about research methodology and methods
YouTube videos	Watch videos about research philosophy such as: Philosophical Assumptions and Worldviews https://youtu.be/VZEEZgk1yJM The Nature of Social Research https://youtu.be/pQ4RAHXtvS0 Complex Research Terminology Simplified: Paradigms, Ontology, Epistemology and Methodology https://youtu.be/8xvpxBVCo0c David James: How to get clear about method, methodology, epistemology and ontology, once and for all https://youtu.be/b83ZfBoQ_Kw

Activities to explore personal ontological and epistemological assumptions

Activities	Practical examples
Discussing philosophical assumptions with others	Justify and explain personal ontological and epistemological assumptions with PhD supervisors Explore philosophical points of view with other postgraduate student peers Ask questions to researchers and review other comments on www.researchgate.net, www.academia.edu, PhD blogs and social media sites
Writing the ontological and epistemological positioning	Keep a reflective journal exploring personal philosophical ideas (in addition to helping to develop and shape a position, this adds to the research audit trail) Include philosophical position in the initial research proposal for organisational and ethical approval

feel trapped in a 'chicken and egg' situation appreciating that learning the research style will come from conducting the study, but some level of understanding about what type of research is still needed to select it at the outset of the research design stage.

When contemplating methodological choices, the researcher can either rule grounded theory in or out by considering that grounded theory research:

- Builds a theory about a topic where little is known or for a subject area which lacks a theoretical basis.
- Seeks to 'explain' and not just 'describe' the phenomenon of interest.
- Is concerned with processes and actions, particularly social processes.

The research questions for my PhD study (Baid, in press)[1] asked: how is sustainability constructed by practitioners working in critical care[2] and what are the social processes involved in making sustainability a component of critical care practice? An initial literature review revealed that no theoretical framework existed to explain sustainability in critical care practice. Grounded theory was partly justified as an appropriate choice then because the topic lacked definition and explanation within the existing published knowledge-base. Other rationalisation for the study to be grounded theory research came from aiming to explain what sustainability in critical care practice meant to people working in critical care (i.e. how they 'construct' this concept). Finally, the emphasis on explaining influential social processes also justified selecting grounded theory for the research design.

Julie Scholes, in Chapter 4, expands on how different people use the phrase 'grounded theory', which some refer to as the methodology and others as the methods. A grounded theory is also the outcome for what the research generates. The original texts focused more on grounded theory to be a collection of procedural tools for the research methods than necessitating a philosophical explanation of background methodology (Glaser & Strauss, 1967; Strauss, 1987). An additional consideration is to use grounded theory methods within other types of research, such as for a case study design (Halaweh, Fidler, & McRobb, 2008). Postgraduate students and novice researchers seeking to differentiate grounded theory terminology related to methodology, method and outcome are advised to read Grounded Theory and Grounded Theorizing (Bryant, 2017). I found it essential to break down the differences between the methodology, approach, methods and output, as indicated in Table 5.2. During the planning, it was also vital to confirm congruence throughout the research process to ensure the methodology, approach and methods all lined up appropriately for the chosen philosophical position.

Rationalising grounded theory methodological choices

There are standard procedures commonly used by all grounded theory approaches as listed in the key methods (Table 5.2.) Primarily, the research generates a theory which is 'grounded' in the emerging ideas from the data and not extant literature or pre-existing notions. Data analysis occurs alongside data generation because data is theoretically sampled based on the analysis of previous data. Coding, categorising and theoretical integration occurs until there is an adequate amount of data to build an explanatory theory (theoretical sufficiency). Chapter 4 expands on the explanation of grounded theory methodology and methods for the three main approaches to grounded theory research.

---

1   PhD supervisors included: Julies Scholes (University of Brighton), Janet Richardson (Plymouth University) and Clair Hebron (University of Brighton).
2   Critical care is hospital-based healthcare for critically ill patients with severe, life-threatening illness or injury. 'Critical care' is an umbrella term integrating intensive and high dependency care into one department.

TABLE 5.2 Grounded theory terminology

Research term	Explanation	Grounded theory research examples
Methodology	Draws on philosophical positioning of the researcher to inform how the research will be conducted by clarifying the ontology, epistemology and other theoretical frameworks influencing the research design	Ontology – realist or relativist Epistemology – positivist, interpretivist or constructivist Other influences – symbolic interactionism, pragmatism, feminism, emancipatory
Grounded theory approach	Type of grounded theory study depending on ontological and epistemological positioning of the researcher	Classic (Glaserian) (Glaser & Strauss, 1967; Glaser, 1992) Straussian (Corbin & Strauss, 2015) Constructivist grounded theory (Charmaz, 2014)
Methods	What type of data collection and analysis procedures will I use to implement this approach and gain the knowledge?	Systematic process of concurrent data collection and analysis, using constant comparison and iteratively moving between induction and deduction. Abduction expresses most likely and plausible explanation of the data. Key grounded theory methods: theoretical sampling, theoretical sensitivity, memoing, coding and categorising, theoretical integration, theoretical sufficiency and theory generation from the data and not pre-conceived ideas.
Output	What its produced from enacting these methods and developing the knowledge?	Increased conceptual understanding, but not yet developed into a theory if theoretical sufficiency not established Substantive grounded theory about a defined subject area Formal grounded theory with increased level of conceptual abstraction, broad scope and applicable to a number of substantive areas

Some grounded theorists believe the researcher should stick to only one grounded theory tradition (e.g. classic, Straussian or constructivist) within a particular study to prevent 'method slurring' and a loss of clarity (Evans, 2013; Breckenridge et al., 2012; Glaser & Holton, 2007). For my doctoral research, I initially planned to solely follow Charmaz's (2014) constructivist grounded theory approach. However, there were points when I faced blocks in analytical thinking, and other techniques were pursued to enhance the abstraction of conceptual ideas. I reflexively considered how and why I 'borrowed' from other approaches ensuring that the research process remained consistent with my philosophical positioning throughout. As such, I viewed additional analytical techniques as enriching, not replacing, the constructivist grounded theory approach. Another rationale is that

96 Heather Baid

the boundaries between the different forms of grounded theory research are blurred (Kenny & Fourie, 2015) and permeable (Apramian et al., 2016) which allows some techniques to complement rather than compete with each other.

An adapted version of Schatzman's (1991) dimensional analysis was one of the procedures used in conjunction with the constructivist grounded theory analytical methods. Dimensional analysis provided a structured way to organise codes (subdimensions) and categories (dimensions) into grids for comparative assessment of the dimension's properties within and between participants.

Table 5.3 illustrates the template used to evaluate interview[3] data, arranged according to the properties of dimensions which surfaced from the initial data analysis.

Each dimensional analysis table included as many rows as there were participants at that point of the study. Similarly, there were as many columns as are needed, depending on the number of properties identified for that particular dimension. Selections of interview data were then inputted into the table if the participant discussed ideas related to that column's property. Codes from the initial coding procedures (e.g. after line-by-line coding and incident-by-incident coding) were the subdimensions listed at the top of each property's column. Interview data were not present for all of the participant rows or the property columns if a participant did not discuss data related relevant subdimensions within a property. However, the absence of data could be a significant consideration noted during the analysis. By presenting short quotations of raw data in this systematic and structured way, a 'birds-eye' view of the dimension's properties provided greater insight into the data and offered new ideas not yet seen. Using quotations from the interviews within the table also ensured the analysis was 'grounded' in the data. Memoing occurred throughout

TABLE 5.3 Dimensional analysis table template

	Dimension:		
Properties:	**Property 1**	**Property 2**	**Property 3**
	Subdimensions related to property1	Subdimensions related to property 2	Subdimensions related to property 3
Participant 1			
Participant 2			
Participant 3			

Property = qualities of the dimension

3 Grounded theory research could potentially collect qualitative or qualitative data, depending on the approach taken and nature of the research question. Commonly, grounded theory research generates qualitative data from interviews, focus groups and direct observation. The doctoral research used 1:1, semi-structured interviews as the main data collection method.

Engaging with grounded theory research   **97**

this dimensionalising process to capture new thoughts, impressions and perceptions gained from the analysis of the comparative table.

A specific example of early dimensional analysis from my doctoral research is provided in Table 5.4, although this is only a part of the table which included a total of 11 rows (for 11 participants) and six columns for further properties of the dimension 'working practices'. There were also other interview quotes placed in the full table with Table 5.4 intended to be a snapshot summary. With this dimension of working practices, stewardship stood out as a significant process and eventually became one of the major categories in the grounded theory. Dimensional analysis, therefore, aided the organisation and evaluation of data, codes and

TABLE 5.4 Dimension table example

Dimension: Working practices		
Properties: **Change**	**Stewardship**	**Teamwork**
• Adapting to change • Accepting change • Being open to change • Facilitating new ways of working • Engaging people with change	• Stewarding – general (appropriate use of critical care services) • Stewarding – financial (appropriate use of money) • Stewarding – environmental (appropriate use of supplies)	• Working together as a team • Team building
Participant 1	*"We can either treat people earlier, or we can prevent inappropriate admissions."*	
Participant 2 *"Changing the culture of how you work is very difficult to do. Unless you have everyone on board with that, it becomes very difficult."*	*"It is about encouraging staff to make sure if you're using a particular type of dressing, some of which are hideously expensive, please make sure you use it appropriately, not just because you think well that looks quite nice."*	*"How do you get people to be in that way of thinking and working together as a team all going in the same place thinking about the longer term."*
Participant 3	*"It's using equipment and the items as, they should be without waste or without opening up things by mistake or there's the whole product wasted, and you've got the packaging to chuck away."*	

Note: This is only a small selection of the original table which included 11 participant rows and 3 other properties of the dimension of working practices (creativity and flexibility, non-technical skills and just-in-case practice).

properties within a category (dimension), which then allowed for further theoretical sampling and progressed the analysis in a focused, data-driven manner.

After all the 11 participants were interviewed, each dimension and sub-dimension were mapped into a summary table for one large view of the key concepts identified in the data. Table 5.5 presents a small part of this summary table to demonstrate the systematic way I compared ideas across all of the participant data. Evaluating if a subject matter was present, absent, discussed but for an action 'not' being done or inconclusive (see legend of Table 5.5) added to the analysis to comprehend more about the relationships, patterns and connections between and within the interview data.

Both dimensional analysis and Straussian grounded theory use a matrix which Corbin and Strauss explain is "an analytic device to help the analyst keep track of the interplay of conditions/consequences and subsequent actions/interactions and to trace their paths of connectivity" (Strauss & Corbin, 1998). In dimensional analysis, Kools et al. (1996) indicate the explanatory matrix highlights the most significant abstract dimension from which all other concepts are centred around (i.e. the core category acting as the data's central organising phenomenon). The dimension's properties are then critiqued and organised according to whether they are context, conditions, processes or consequences:

- *Context* – background, nature and details about the substantive area of the research to put boundaries around the inquiry.
- *Conditions* – things which influence actions by hindering, promoting or moulding in some way.
- *Processes* – actions as a result of the conditions which can be deliberate, purposeful and calculated or unintentional, involuntary and inadvertent.
- *Consequences* – the end result of the actions identified as processes.

Similarly, the Straussian conditional/consequential matrix focused on the context, conditions and consequences of the most significant, higher level, abstract concept to form links between micro and macro conditions impacting on this central category (Corbin & Strauss, 2015). It took numerous rounds of auditioning different concepts as the central idea in the matrix before one particular category stood out as holding the most explanatory power. This core idea that stood out as having the most 'fit' and centrality was a decision-making process called satisficing. Grounded theory analysis borrows the language of existing theories to explain the data gathered for the current study. The concept of satisficing came from business literature, which is when someone is 'satisfied' they have reached a goal while 'sufficing' within the resources available (Simon, 1957, 1997). Other major categories tried out but rejected as the central organising phenomenon included the concepts of stewarding and bounded rationality. However, these concepts still held importance in explaining some aspects of the topic of sustainability in critical care practice, which justified including them as supporting categories in the final grounded theory.

TABLE 5.5 Dimensional analysis summary table example

Category (Dimension)	Codes (Subdimensions)	P01	P02	P03	P04
Sustainability definition	Environmental sustainability	Image Picture 137.png	Image Picture 238.png	Image Picture 237.png	Image Picture 236.png
	Financial sustainability	Image Picture 141.png	Image Picture 256.png	Image Picture 381.png	Image Picture 390.png
	Social sustainability	Image Picture 164.png	Image Picture 607.png	O	O
	Sustaining critical care as a service	O	O	O	Image Picture 446.png
	Unclear on meaning of sustainability	O	Image Picture 170.png	O	O
	Linking types of sustainability together	Image Picture 172.png	Image Picture 293.png	Image Picture 383.png	Image Picture 430.png
	Negative connotation to sustainability	O	Image Picture 292.png	O	O
Communication	Multi-disciplinary team	Image Picture 524.png	O	Image Picture 216.png	Image Picture 407.png
	Negotiating care	Image Picture 526.png	O	O	Image Picture 409.png
	Trust wide generic emails	O	Image Picture 246.png	Image Picture 315.png	Image Picture 408.png
	Discuss sustainability in critical care	Image Picture 183.png	X	X	X

Category (Dimension)	Codes (Subdimensions)	P01	P02	P03	P04
Values and beliefs	Valuing sustainability as important	Image Picture 527.png	Image Picture 297.png	Image Picture 384.png	Image Picture 410.png
	Tension between own values and reality	Image Picture 541.png	Image Picture 245.png	?	O
	Changing culture of practice	Image Picture 547.png	Image Picture 290.png	Image Picture 220.png	O
	Values, beliefs, attitudes	Image Picture 569.png	Image Picture 291.png	O	O

Legend:

Image Picture 630.png	**Present in the data**	Concept directly discussed by participant in the interview
O	**Absent in the data**	Concept not discussed by participant in the interview
X	**Negative data**	Concept discussed but as 'not' being present (e.g. recycling is mentioned but in relation to recycling not being done)
?	**Inconclusive**	Unclear during data analysis with further clarification required

Note: This is only a small selection of the original table which included 11 participant columns and numerous other dimensions and subdimensions within the rows.

Engaging with grounded theory research   **101**

There is minimal literature on dimensional analysis, and that which exists is quite old (Schatzman & Strauss, 1973; Schatzman, 1991; Gilgun, 1993; Bowers & Schatzman, 2009). However, I additionally learned about adding in dimensional analysis and Straussian principles to the constructivist grounded theory analytical procedures through the oral tradition of learning from PhD supervisors and reading other doctoral theses (Petty, 2009; Nixon, 2013; Smith, 2013; Trapani, 2014; Wallis, 2014; Hassall, 2016). The flexibility of grounded theory facilitated this mixing of different approaches, allowing me to adapt and modify the analytical process as the data analysis progressed. I then found a way which best suited my ability to extract, organise and explain relevant abstract concepts in the data, all the while maintaining consistency with the constructivist philosophical positioning.

Some of my postgraduate student peers, also undertaking grounded theory research, found dimensional analysis to be constraining and impeded rather than helped their data analysis. They found the dimensional analysis techniques unhelpful, which for them, felt forced and unnatural to try and put data into boxes. My experience was quite the opposite. It was dimensional analysis and the Straussian conditional/consequential matrix techniques which liberated my analytical thinking at a point of stagnation during the focused coding stage of Charmaz's (2014) grounded theory approach. Therefore, I am rationalising my methodological choices to explain what worked for this particular piece of research. Novice researchers can find their personal style by trying out various data analysis tools, techniques and aids, or staying true to one particular approach, as best suits them.

Another analytical tool borrowed from the Straussian grounded theory approach was that of writing a storyline (Corbin & Strauss, 2015). As the 'story of the case', a storyline takes the form on an extended theoretical memo explaining the developing theory once theoretical integration brings together a central concept and other major categories. Telling a story helps to make sense of something. Stories convey messages, bring abstract ideas into practical understanding and provide a way of communicating concepts to other people. My storyline, therefore, enabled me to find meaning in the rationale for the selected central organising phenomenon. Furthermore, the storyline became the foundation for the PhD thesis findings chapter as an initial scaffolding to explain the large quantities of qualitative data produced from the interviews.

Finally, the storyline also became an output as a draft summary of the early theory, which I could then share with supervisors and participants. Revealing the storyline to my supervisors provided the opportunity to articulate and justify theoretical integration and added to the audit trail evidence for 'how' the research process unfolded. Sending the summarised version of the storyline to participants was one of the ways member checking occurred. Birt et al.'s (2016) 'Synthesised Member Checking' (SMC) technique was followed whereby participants could read the summarised storyline before a second interview. In this follow-up contact with participants, very focused questions explored whether the theory explained in the storyline resonated with their experiences. The participants confirmed that the proposed theory made sense to them and provided examples for how it could pragmatically work if applied to clinical practice. Thus, member checking facilitated co-construction (in keeping with a constructivist grounded theory approach) and provided further evidence for theoretical sufficiency. Had the participants not been able to see value or relevance of the auditioning theory, I would have then had a sense for how to theoretically sample new data.

There is a debate in both grounded theory and qualitative research literature about whether this type of member checking is beneficial or a hindrance within the research methods. Researchers who are critical (Sandelowski, 1993; Glaser, 2002, 2007; Morse, 2015) argue that member checking becomes problematic because the participants might:

- Be unable to interpret abstract concepts if they lack analytical research skills.
- Disagree with the analysed data.
- Not remember the points they made during the first contact.
- Change their views which then conflicts with their previous ideas.
- View repeated contact with a researcher as meddling, interfering and intrusive.

I took a relativist, constructivist position for the doctoral research though, which embraces subjectivity, recognises people's views will not remain static and values collaborating and co-building theory with the participants (Koelsch, 2013). I viewed member checking as a positive element of the research methods then because it facilitated power-sharing with participants and contributed to the verification of theoretical sufficiency (Charmaz, 2014). Reflexivity within memoing before, during and after member checking allowed me to stay aware of the potential limitations and to confirm methodological congruence in returning to the same participants. Moreover, I anticipated and reflected on what I would have done had any of member checking's disadvantages prominently impeded on the research process. Memoing after comparing each participant's first and second interview data revealed that some of the specific examples differed, but the underpinning abstract concepts of the central organising phenomenon and other major categories remained consistent, adding credibility to the proposed grounded theory.

Conducting grounded theory research as a postgraduate student

I was a novice grounded theorist at the beginning of the doctoral study. Julie Scholes, in Chapter 6, encourages new researchers to trust the method and the process and the learning will come. Having completed the project and defended the thesis, I am increasingly confident in my knowledge and practice with conducting constructivist grounded theory research, which only came from experiential 'doing'. This section will now offer pragmatic and practical advice for those who are new to grounded theory. I will include things I wish I had known more about at the beginning of my doctoral research, along with aspects of my learning which were particularly valuable while undertaking this type of research as a postgraduate student.

Write, write, write

Writing memos is an essential component of any grounded theory research process, regardless of the philosophical positioning and approach. I memoed throughout the planning, implementation and evaluation of the research which provided an extensive memo bank of unedited thoughts, perceptions, feelings and impressions. In grounded theory research, the memos become another source of data. As such, memos are presented in the findings chapter to supplement other sources of data. Birks, Chapman, and Francis (2008) encapsulate the purpose of memoing with the abbreviation MEMO: **M**apping research activities, **E**xtracting meaning from data, **M**aintaining momentum and **O**pening communication.

For me, writing in memos held great importance in explaining the what, how and why of both the research process and analytical thinking during the theory development. Every researcher will have their style for how memos are written, collated and stored. The essential thing is to write. Memoing enhances creativity, frees up blocks if 'analytic paralysis' impedes the data analysis and provides a safe space to take risks while exploring meaning found in the data (Charmaz, 2014; Birks & Mills, 2015). I found it helpful to differentiate the memos according to their type which could be dated and cross-referenced. This coding system organised the documentation for how the grounded theory developed and enabled me to quickly find memos related to analysis and theory development in the latter stages when reviewing memos served key to theoretical integration. Filing the memos according to their type also made it easier and more efficient to pick out different ones to use within the methods and findings chapters of the final thesis. The various kinds of memos I kept included:

- RES – research memo about the methods and process of conducting a grounded theory study.
- DEV – development memo about the personal and professional development of myself as a newly developing researcher. This memoing complemented the research (RES) memos but focused more on how I progressed within the domains of the *Vitae Researcher Development Framework* (RDF)[4]
- OPE – operational memo about logistical information related to activities throughout planning and implementation of the project (these were kept within an ongoing table which also provided a clear audit trail of research activities).
- SAM – sampling memo with an emphasis on theoretical sampling.

---

4   The *Vitae Researcher Development Framework (RDF)* provides postgraduate students with a structured planner for designing and evaluating personal development as a new researcher. The RDF is based on these four domains about successful researcher characteristics: (1) Knowledge and intellectual abilities; (2) Personal effectiveness; (3) Research governance and organisation; and (4) Engagement, influence and impact. The RDF is freely available to postgraduate students on the Vitae website: www.vitae.ac.uk/researchers-professional-development

- REF – reflective / reflexive memo.
- DAT – data collection memo about how data was generated.
- ANA – analytical memo about the data analysis ideas, breakthroughs and decisions.
- COD – coding memo about codes emerging from the initial coding procedures.
- CAT – category memo about coding the codes to explain high-level concepts and abstraction.
- THE – theory memo in the later analysis stages exploring theoretical integration and auditioning of the central organising phenomenon.

Grounded theory research aims to generate an explanatory theory which focuses on processes and actions. It is then beneficial to write codes as a gerund (verb ending in 'ing'). Initial coding for the first time is challenging. At first, I simply rephrased the points made by the participant described the data and did not move the explanation forward. Reminders about 'where is the ing' prompted more in-depth exploration about meaning related to actions, which subsequently transitioned my analytical thinking into a higher level of conceptual abstraction. According to Charmaz (2014, p. 124), "coding with gerunds and studying processes enables you to discern implicit connections – and, simultaneously, gives you control over your data and emerging analysis."

Data collection involving 1:1 or focused group interviews typically uses an audio recorder to document the conversation and supplemented by the researcher taking notes. Experienced researchers may not transcribe, or they might choose to not audio record at all. The expert grounded theorist could have the listening and analytical skills to pick out abstract concepts without the need for recording and transcribing data. For myself as a novice researcher, recording was essential because I could then go back and listen again which enhanced my ability to analyse the data. I chose not to have someone else transcribe the interviews though. During manual transcribing, I reflected on the meaning of what I typed and concurrently memoed to authenticate my reasoning throughout this data analysis.

Administration skills

Postgraduate students have an enormous learning curve to face due to the amount of new knowledge needed to plan, implement and evaluate their research study. Additionally, I found it necessary to improve my computer skills for the administration of the project. I experientially learned these skills along the way of conducting the study, although I could have saved vast amounts of time if I had developed a more robust understanding of practical information and technology skills from the outset.

I would recommend postgraduate students consider the 'top-tips' listed in Table 5.6 for practical Microsoft Office Word document skills to be more efficient in the administration aspect of conducting grounded theory research. The ability to

Engaging with grounded theory research **105**

effectively use extra functions within Word was particularly important during the writing up phase of preparing the final thesis. Grounded theory research feels like a 4D process, making it difficult to present a linear report when the project involves multiple iterative and concurrent activities. The Word document skills in Table 5.6 can address this difficulty as learned through the help function within Word itself or the Microsoft website for videos, support and online training (https://support. office.com/en-gb/word). Investing a small amount of time into this type of Office Word knowledge and skill will save large quantities of time later on. Taking advantage of all the higher-level functions within Word also facilitates the final thesis or report produced from the research to be accurate, polished and publishable.

Some researchers use qualitative data analysis software to assist with organising and analysing the data. I chose not to use this type of software and instead manually sorted, arranged and stored the interview data and memos myself. My rationales were that I felt a manual process would be best as my first grounded theory piece of research to stay as close to the data as possible and to not get lost in the learning of how to use the software. I also recognised that the actual critical thinking comes from the researcher, not the software. I did not want to inadvertently allow the computer programme to impede my analysis as a novice researcher. The use of qualitative data analysis software is then a personal preference depending on the style, nature and context of the project. Birks and Mills (2015) offer guidance and examples of when and how software is beneficial to grounded theory data analysis.

While manually transcribing the interview data, I did find it useful though to use keyboard shortcuts for pausing, replaying and rewinding the audio recorder. I found this to be more efficient and user-friendly compared to a foot-pedal or transcription software. The actual buttons to press for the hotkey shortcuts will depend on the computer (e.g. some computers have these functions built in on the 'F' buttons at the top of the keyboard) or audio player (search for the hotkeys built into that app or playing software).

Support from others

Grounded theory research can be very rewarding, but it is also challenging, time-consuming and complex to learn as a postgraduate student researching a novice. Seek out support from other people to discuss your questions, hear similar experiences and receive feedback on how to develop your project. I found it beneficial to meet regularly with my student peer group of other MSc and PhD students conducting grounded theory research. A local grounded theory special interest group in the University not only provided lectures and workshops on learning the craft of grounded theory but also offered valuable networking and discussion time. Finally, look for support via social media, such as with grounded theory Facebook groups and Twitter handles.

106 Heather Baid

TABLE 5.6 Microsoft Office Word skills to help postgraduate students

Function (Microsoft, 2019)	Explanation
Ctrl – Alt – Z	Grounded theory reporting requires frequently going back and forth between different sections of a large Word document file. Pressing **Ctrl – Alt – Z** buttons all at the same time takes you back to the last place you were typing.
Quick navigation	The navigation pane appears if you press **Ctrl – F** at the same time. Use the **font styles for headings** throughout the document to have them presented in the navigation pane hyperlinks. You can also use the **search document** box to look for a word or phrase (listed under **results)**.
Searching within multiple Word files	Follow these steps to search for a word/phrase within multiple files in a folder: Open folder > **View** tab > **Options** > **Change folder and search options** > **Search** > **Always search file names and contents**. Searching within multiple Word files is useful while manually looking for terms, codes and categories during comparative data analysis.
Cross-referencing	The **insert caption function** in the **references tab** labels tables and figures in numerical order. Create **Bookmarks** through these steps: Highlight the word/phrase which you want to bookmark > Insert tab > Links > Bookmark. Use the **cross-reference function** to refer to the label/page number of a table, figure or bookmark. If the **font styles for headings** are used for headings and subheadings, you can also use the **cross-reference function** to insert a **numbered item,** choosing the paragraph number/page number. In the **references tab**, use the **Table of Contents** function to build automatic lists of headings, tables and figures.
Updating fields	**Cross-referencing** puts a bookmark, table, figure or the page number in a **field – Ctrl + clicking** on the field jumps straight to that place in the document. At the end, **right click** on the **field** and manually **Update Field** to ensure the correct label or page number remains. Alternatively, press **Ctrl – A** at the same time to **select all**, then click on the **F9 button** to **update all fields** in the document.
Footnotes	**Footnotes** within the findings chapter can refer to published literature or other sections of the document to be transparent about theoretically sampled literature (and therefore not forced as pre-conceived ideas). **Footnotes** also help to make links between overlapping content within the document. The **insert footnote function** sits in the **References tab**. The findings footnotes can include a short explanation for why a publication, personal reflection or other prompts acted as conceptual levers for further data collection and analysis. This type of footnote also serves as a memo within the thesis/report itself and adds to the audit trail for how the theory developed.

Transitioning into an early career researcher

Grounded theory research theoretically ends when there is a point of theoretical sufficiency, i.e. once there is enough data for developing an explanatory theory about important processes related to the phenomenon of the study. However, over time, the context, conditions and consequences could shift, and other new data may become available which further strengthens or influences the theory. In that respect, grounded theory research could be viewed as an everlasting project. Glaser and Strauss (1967, p. 40) advise that "the published word is not the final one, but only a pause in the never-ending process of generating theory." Similarly, Saunders et al. (2018, p. 1901) state that theoretical sufficiency is "an ongoing, cumulative judgment that one makes, and perhaps never completes, rather than something that can be pinpointed at a specific juncture."

For the postgraduate student, there are time restrictions on when to complete the research which may not be enough for verifying full theoretical sufficiency. It can be helpful to view theoretical sufficiency as a continuum though which begins with an initial proposal and becomes enhanced with ongoing development and verification. It may not be feasible for a postgraduate MSc or PhD study to produce a grounded theory with the justification of reaching theoretical sufficiency. One perspective is that instead of using the phrase 'theoretical saturation' as presented in some grounded theory literature (Glaser & Strauss, 1967), consider the implications for 'sufficiency' which implies adequacy, not maximal fullness. It is also beneficial not to feel the pressure to produce a completed grounded theory because that may not be feasible within the timeframe of the postgraduate course submission deadline. The final thesis/research report could present the initial framework for conceptual ideas that may lead to a grounded theory with further theoretical sampling and added data. However, the formation of the grounded theory would then occur after the timeframe of the university course project. For my doctoral study, I rationalised an initial level of theoretical sufficiency, but further development of this substantive theory is planned as an early career researcher, including testing out the theory's practical application.

This chapter told the story of my journey as a doctoral student engaging with grounded theory research for the first time as a novice. Sharing these experiences and learning points gained from the project is intended to help other postgraduate students considering grounded theory as a methodology, method or outcome for their own research.

References

Apramian, T., S. Cristancho, C. Watling, and L. Lingard. 2016. (Re)grounding grounded theory: A close reading of theory in four schools. *Qualitative Research*, 17(4): 359–376.

Baid, H. 2019. Sustainability in critical care practice: A constructivist grounded theory [Online]. Brighton: University of Brighton. Available from https://research.brighton.ac.uk/en/publications/satisficing-for-sustainability-in-critical-care-practice-a-constr

Birks, M., Y. Chapman, and K. Francis. 2008. Memoing in qualitative research: Probing data and processes. *Journal of Research in Nursing*, 13(1): 68–75.

Birks, M., and J. Mills. 2015. *Grounded theory: A practical guide* (2nd ed.). London: SAGE.

Birt, L., S. Scott, D. Cavers, C. Campbell, and F. Walter. 2016. Member checking a tool to enhance trustworthiness or merely a nod to validation? *Qualitative Health Research*, 26(13): 1802–1811. doi:10.1177/1049732316654870

108 Heather Baid

Bowers, B., and L. Schatzman. 2009. Dimensional analysis. In *Developing grounded theory: The second generation*, edited by J.M. Morse, P.N. Stern, J. Corbin, B. Bowers, *et al.* Walnut Creek, CA: Left Coast Press.

Breckenridge, J., D. Jones, I. Elliott, and M. Nicol. 2012. Choosing a methodological path: Reflections on the constructivist turn. *Grounded Theory Review*, 11(1): 64–71.

Bryant, A. 2017. *Grounded theory and grounded theorizing: Pragmatism in research practice.* New York, NY: Oxford University Press.

Charmaz, K. 2014. *Constructing grounded theory.* London: SAGE.

Corbin, J.M., and A.L. Strauss. 2015. *Basics of qualitative research: Techniques and procedures for developing grounded theory* (4th ed.). Los Angeles: SAGE.

Evans, G.L. 2013. A novice researcher's first walk through the maze of grounded theory. *Grounded Theory Review*, 12(1): 37–55.

Gilgun, J. 1993. Dimensional analysis and grounded theory: Interviews with Leonard Schatzman. *Qualitative Family Research*, 7(1 & 2): 1–7.

Glaser, B.G. 1992. *Basics of grounded theory analysis: Emergence vs forcing.* Mill Valley, CA: Sociology Press.

Glaser, B.G. 2002. Conceptualization: On theory and theorizing using grounded theory. *International Journal of Qualitative Methods*, 1(2): 23–38.

Glaser, B.G. 2007. Naturalist inquiry and grounded theory. *Historical Social Research/Historische Sozialforschung (Supplement)*, 3(3): 114–132.

Glaser, B.G., and J. Holton. 2007. Remodeling grounded theory. *Historical Social Research/Historische Sozialforschung*, 19: 47–68.

Glaser, B.G., and A.L. Strauss. 1967. *The discovery of grounded theory: Strategies for qualitative research.* New York, NY: Aldine de Gruyter.

Halaweh, M., C. Fidler, and S. McRobb. 2008. Integrating the grounded theory method and case study research methodology within is research: A possible 'road map'. *ICIS 2008 Proceedings*. 29th International Conference on Information Systems, Paris. Available from https://aisel.aisnet.org/cgi/viewcontent.cgi?article=1052&context=icis2008

Hassall, J.L. 2016. *Women's decisions to exercise in pregnancy: Negotiating conflicting identities* (Unpublished doctoral thesis). University of Brighton, UK.

Kenny, M., and R. Fourie. 2015. Contrasting classic, Straussian, and constructivist grounded theory: Methodological and philosophical conflicts. *The Qualitative Report*, 20(8): 1270.

Koelsch, L.E. 2013. Reconceptualizing the member check interview. *International Journal of Qualitative Methods*, 12(1): 168–179.

Kools, S., M. McCarthy, R. Durham, and L. Robrecht. 1996. Dimensional analysis: Broadening the conception of grounded theory. *Qualitative Health Research*, 6(3): 312–330.

Microsoft. 2019. *Welcome to Office help and training.* Microsoft. [Online]. Available from https://support.office.com/ [12 May 2019]

Morse, J.M. 2015. Critical analysis of strategies for determining rigor in qualitative inquiry. *Qualitative Health Research*, 25(9): 1212–1222.

Nixon, E. 2013. *Healthy-illness representation of HIV in the UK* (Unpublished doctoral thesis). University of Brighton, UK.

O'Leary, Z. 2017. *The essential guide to doing your research project* (3rd ed.). Thousand Oaks, CA: SAGE.

Petty, N.J. 2009. Towards clinical expertise: Learning transitions of neuromusculoskeletal physiotherapists (Unpublished doctoral thesis). University of Brighton, Brighton.

Sandelowski, M. 1993. Rigor or rigor mortis: The problem of rigor in qualitative research revisted. *Advances in Nursing Science*, 16(2): 1–8.

Saunders, B., J. Sim, T. Kingstone, S. Baker, J. Waterfield, B. Bartlam, H. Burroughs, and C. Jinks. 2018. Saturation in qualitative research: Exploring its conceptualization and operationalization. *Quality & Quantity*, 52(4): 1893–1907.

Schatzman, L. 1991. Dimensional analysis: Notes on an alternative approach to the grounding of theory in qualitative research. In *Social organization and social process: Essays in honor of anselm strauss*, edited by D.R. Maines. New York: Walter de Gruyter.

Schatzman, L., and A.L. Strauss. 1973. *Field research: Strategies for a natural sociology*. Englewood Cliffs, NJ: Prentice Hall.

Simon, H.A. 1957. *Models of man. Social and rational. Mathematical essays on rational human behavior in a social setting*. New York: John Wiley & Sons.

Simon, H.A. 1997. *Administrative behavior: A study of decision-making processes in administrative organizations* (4th ed.). New York: The Free Press.

Smith, S.A. 2013. *Decision-making in acute care nursing with deteriorating patients* (Unpublished doctoral thesis). University of Brighton, UK.

Strauss, A.L. 1987. *Qualitative analysis for social scientists*. Cambridge: Cambridge University Press.

Strauss, A.L., and J.M. Corbin. 1998. *Basics of qualitative research: Techniques and procedures for developing grounded theory* (2nd ed.). Thousand Oaks, CA: SAGE.

Trapani, J. 2014. Referring in critical care: nurses as dual agents (Unpublished doctoral thesis). University of Brighton, UK.

Wallis, J. 2014. *Emotional demands of learning to become a teacher: Trainee PE teacher experiences of confronting problematic situations* (Unpublished doctoral thesis). University of Brighton, UK.

6

FROM PHENOMENOLOGY TO PRACTICE

Theoretical foundations and phenomenological methods

Kate Galvin, Oliver Thurlow and Rebecca Player

Phenomenology rests on and is informed by a long and deep philosophical heritage, and while the application of phenomenology and its implications have been evident in a wide range of disciplines in the human sciences – for example in psychology (Giorgi, 2009), in philosophy of medicine, with an embodiment focus (Leder, 1990), in occupational therapy (Fitzpatrick & Finlay, 2008), in nursing (Dahlberg, Dahlberg, & Nystrom, 2008), and in education (Saevi & Fornan, 2014), to name just a few – and it continues to develop and pursue new theoretical and empirical directions. This chapter outlines some distinctions about phenomenology setting it apart from other qualitative methods by offering some ways of defining what a phenomenological approach is and what this means in the pursuit of enquiry. We illustrate how the philosophical considerations of a phenomenological approach can be translated into specific methods and procedures for carrying out research in the human sciences, specifically making a case for descriptive phenomenological enquiry (because most general qualitative research methods text do not offer this specific emphasis). The chapter briefly acknowledges philosophical foundations and heritage but we refer readers to Chapter Seven (Graham Stew) in this volume, and important sources such as Moran (2000), Zahavi (2019), and Spiegelberg (1994) that fully elucidate the vital philosophical ground that has been developing for over 100 years. The key focus we draw on for the purpose of this present chapter is how a foundation laid by Husserl offers us firstly a way to use 'the life-world'[1] as a source of knowledge. The lifeworld *is the ground* for enquiry. Secondly an emphasis that is not focused on articulating theory, but is instead, a beneficial way of describing the *whatness* or *quiddity* of a phenomenon *as it appears*. The overall purpose of such an approach is to more deeply understand the phenomenon and its essential features.

---

1   The 'lifeworld' refers to our seamless experience of the stream of experiential happenings which are all in relation, these relationships are in time, in space, in body and with others and are intertwined.

Phenomenology as method

A prominent author on the subject and historical development of phenomenology is Herbert Spiegelberg (1904–1990). An American philosopher, Spiegelberg was a strong proponent of phenomenology and its historical body of character. Spiegelberg (1994) asserts the challenge to reductionism that phenomenology poses. In his 1994 *Introduction to the History of Phenomenology*, Spiegelberg describes the positivistic quest for reductionism as a "bulldozer" (p. 608) which denies the richness and meanings associated with experiential phenomena, and in turn oversimplifies our shared experiences through statistical measurement. Placing phenomenology at the centre of reclaiming the depth that is required for understanding immediate experience, Spiegelberg (1994) is insistent on the nature of application of method, outlining the three essential steps of 'investigating particular phenomena, investigating general essences, and apprehending essential relationships among essences' as crucial if one is to uncover overlooked insights about a phenomenon. Giorgi (2009) offers a specific definitional boundary for phenomenological research that draws on Husserl's philosophy and provides criteria by which to judge the phenomenological nature of a study. These include a consideration of essences, intentionality, lifeworld, intuition, phenomenological reduction and imaginative variation. These criteria are now unfolded in the context of discussing the application of phenomenological stance to empirical research work. Considered to be a Husserlian approach to phenomenology, science, and psychology, Amedeo Giorgi's Duquesne school of descriptive phenomenology is considered to be a rigorous and systematic approach to applied phenomenology. Staying close to Husserl's effort of developing a scientific strategy for philosophy, Giorgi (2009) sought to develop a method that would respect the investigation of psychological phenomena that would equal that of the reductionistic methods he had previously been trained in. Critiquing the control of environmental conditions in applied research, Giorgi (2009) respects the subjective and qualitative factors that are present in the individual lifeworld. Moreover, Giorgi's phenomenology is a commitment to human reality, whereby human psychology can become its own discipline, as opposed to mainstream psychology which, Giorgi (2009) claims, has followed the philosophical and methodological frameworks of the natural sciences. Further, Giorgi (2009) has critiqued the method and setting in which humans and animals have been studied, with both of these facing a distorted reality in a way that would not produce the same behaviour in a naturalistic enquiry.

Furthermore, the positivistic, reductionist research design relies heavily on a laboratory-based context to study phenomena of the world. The laboratory is often associated with removal of context and control of variables with experimental procedures that offer causal 'laws and facts' regarding phenomena from microbiological organisms to human stimulus-response. However, Giorgi (2009) importantly identifies the inherent flaw of attempting to understand the psychology of human experience within a laboratory setting, as the variety of contexts usually attached to an experience have significant and important implications on *the meaning*. Though discussed briefly, Giorgi (2009, p. 115) underscores the necessity of understanding the context or situated position in which the human "stream of consciousness" (experience) is exposed to outside of conditions that can easily be controlled or repeated. For instance, Broome's (2011) descriptive phenomenological study of police officers using deadly force while on duty is a sufficient example of the importance of meaning in a context that is not pre-controlled. Broome (2011, pp. 77–78) addresses the complications of context by suggesting "it is the plucking out of the psychological phenomenon (along with the person in whom it is inherently found) from its natural habitat and forcing it into the contrived context that imposes the greatest threats of 'contaminating' it prior to its analysis and subsequent understanding". It is however important to note that Giorgi (2009) is careful to acknowledge that a researcher must be pragmatic in their research projects. One has to be directed toward the demand of the research question, rather than employing a methodology out of past experience that generated a particular liking.

For the purpose of this chapter, taking a beginning point influenced by Giorgi (2009; Giorgi, Giorgi, & Morley, 2017) we would like to suggest some stages of phenomenological research as a scientific practice that is informed by phenomenological philosophy.

1. An articulation and delineation of experiential phenomena that are of interest in the phenomenological research study. This is an essential first step, to clearly articulate the phenomenon under study. This step is much more complex than it may first seem and requires reflection and thoughtfulness.
2. Collecting descriptions and concrete examples of others' experiences that are situated occurrences of the phenomenon. An example question of participants here would be: can you describe in as much detail as possible a situation in which [the experience] occurred? This is followed by collection of many examples of aspects of the lifeworld from the participant.
3. Reflecting and intuiting to illicit the meanings of such experiences. Here there is a slowing down in a mode of reflection, capturing description of essential meanings of the phenomena that are nuanced rather than absolutes, experiential happenings are studied and fresh insights can emerge from 'the details'.
4. Formulating a narrative structure that highlights essential meanings across cases. This offers a written understanding of the nature of the phenomenon that cares for how the phenomenon coheres through all its variations (the whole) as well as illustrating how its parts (variations) help make sense of the whole. In other words, how the constituent parts make sense of the whole phenomenon: what the essential features of a phenomenon that cohere through all its variations are. The aim here is to arrive at an account of transferable meanings or in more technical language, pointing to constituents of the meaning that characterise the phenomena, sometimes called essences.

Drawing on Husserl, descriptive phenomenology would claim that the potential depth and detail of the meaning of a descriptive account of an experience can easily go beyond the individual's (whom is having the experience) judgement and inference.

From phenomenology to practice **113**

Human phenomenon that people live with and through do have some generalizable properties – for example there is something about the experience of human well-being, or the human experiences of dignity, anger, joy, sorrow, that we can recognise in the descriptions from different individuals and there is also something about the properties of these phenomenon that tell us that there is something distinctive about well-being, dignity, anger, joy, sorrow: we recognise them as real experiences. Researchers as human beings participate in the world, more specifically we participate in *the lifeworld*, in part or in whole, and as such we have the potential to know something and understand what these might be like experientially. Therefore, a description of a situated experience can lead to more insights that are transferable and which can deepen understanding of the phenomenon under investigation These insights can constitute a pattern that connects a number of experiential examples or variations. In other words, the descriptions that our participants share with us are not experienced as hollow or meaningless words given to us by others', instead we already have how text and words point to a whole world of significance. As human researchers in a shared lifeworld we can reflect on the experiential world of such significances and seek to substantiate if these experiential significances are confirmed by the details and varieties of an experience described to us in the text. There is an important point here that is to do with how phenomenology is not focused on representation or mere reports, or in presenting the 'voices' of participants in similar or other words arranged as themes. Instead the descriptive phenomenological analysis quest is to move beyond the words of participants to illicit meanings in a more general way, here the experience is *an entry point* or portal to transferable meanings that *can clarify the phenomena under investigation*. Several writers in phenomenology have recommended some stages of analysis that support a disciplined way of intuiting general meanings which are faithful and stay close to the details in descriptive accounts of experiences (Todres & Holloway, 2004; Wertz et al., 2011). It is a process of going back and forth between the details in the descriptions and the phenomenon as it emerges. There is a form of discipline in staying close to the details but at the same time engaging in a particular kind of openness to the phenomenon, one which can draw on reflection and imagination. Dahlberg et al. (2008) offer a way of engaging in this form of analysis in their Reflective Lifeworld Research process, and have coined the word 'bridling' to describe a kind of holding back but also a kind of openness at the same time with the overall aim of presenting what is typical of the phenomenon and in offering essences, or what is sometimes called a general structure of the phenomenon. See also Dahlberg and Dahlberg (2003).

Husserl's emphasis on essences has been contested in the phenomenological methods literature and commonly it is argued that it is impossible to provide essences, with arguments about the level of generality and universal applicability that can be achieved. Often it is recommended therefore that an interpretive approach would be a better way forward to respond to this critique. We do not agree that a descriptive phenomenological approach should be cast aside so quickly, as the split between interpretative and descriptive phenomenology has been muddy and is often over emphasised in the qualitative literature. Generally, phenomenology has been divided into two kinds, descriptive and interpretive, with descriptive approach staying close to

Husserl and interpretive close to Heidegger, Gadamer and other key continental philosophers. Interpretive and hermeneutic phenomenologists do not believe that researchers can be successful in suspending their preconceptions, and that researchers can make use of preconceptions productively and demonstrating this explicitly through reflective accounts. This has sometimes been criticised as being too subjective. Hermeneutic phenomenologists also wish to privilege uniqueness and diversity over common essences. However, we think that these distinctions are commonly over-emphasised because both kinds of phenomenology share some common characteristics, they both start in the lifeworld and make use of seamless lifeworld descriptions, rather than 'data' which is more fragmented; they both employ the use of a sensitising reflective analytic approach or the use of bracketing and arrive at a 'fusion of horizons' or an 'essential description' of an *experienced* phenomena. Further, research that aims to apprehend an experienced phenomenon can successfully point *to the bare bones* of the phenomenon, and it is therefore possible to develop a general structure of a phenomenon following phenomenological analysis. The nature of what is precisely meant by 'essence' has sometimes been misunderstood in our view, contributing to this contentious debate. Husserl has provided us with various levels of generality that are possible to achieve, and the literature is replete with examples of essential descriptions of phenomena that offer new understandings (for example, the experience of falling ill with diabetes) (Johansson, Ekeberg, & Dahlberg, 2009); the relatives experience of patients who have undergone 'fast track' surgery with very early discharge (Norlyk & Martinsen, 2013). For a very helpful robust and informative account of the nature of essences and what they are precisely in the context of phenomenological research we refer readers to Dahlberg (2009), where she explores the characteristics of essences in the search for meaning structures in the light of Husserl's ideas on intentionality.

By way of further illustration, the following studies provide general meaning structures that insightfully point to the depth and detail of the phenomenon under study.

Vuoskoski, P. (2014). *Work-Placement Assessment as a Lived-Through Educationally Meaningful Experience of the Student: An Application of the Phenomenological Descriptive Approach.*

> In this study, a phenomenological descriptive method was applied to the clarification of the lived-through educationally meaningful experience in student assessment, related to a work-placement and higher educational context. As an account for an essential structural description is generating scientific knowledge, the study increases understanding of the phenomenon of interest by giving insight into the direct assessment experience and its key constituents, using verbal expressions and acts of consciousness as the medium for accessing the situation of the other, and describing it exactly as experienced as a presence for the experiencer, from an educational perspective.
>
> The Phenomenological analysis of the data showed that a distinguishable chain of events could be discerned, that the participants of the study identified

positively and/or negatively meaningful experiences in assessment, carrying a great deal of personal and educational significance for the student. What constitutes the most essential aspect of living through the educationally meaningful experience in work-placement assessment, in this study, is the intention of the student to obtain self-knowledge through assessment encounters, and the sense of fulfilment of that subjective self-interest. Once the awareness of the self-interest is awakened in the student, the other necessary constituents become possible. These were discovered to be: resemblance of assumptions and practice, sense of shared interest/s, reliance on self and others, sense of safety and openness, sense of emotional engagement, sense of enhancement and support, and challenge to assumptions and self-interest.

(pp. 5–6)

Dahlberg et al. (2009) offers an illustration of the phenomenon of loneliness based on a reflective lifeworld study.

Twenty-six interviews were analysed for meaning with the aim of describing an essential structure for the phenomenon, showing what loneliness is. The analysis shows that the phenomenon of loneliness stands out in meaning as "figure" against a "background" of fellowship, connectedness and context. One is lonely when important others are not there, because either one has rejected them or they have chosen to be rejected and left the person behind, feeling lonely. One can reject others in favour of another kind of connectedness. Such loneliness is restful and pleasant. It involves the lack of tangible context that other present people can offer, yet a context is not missing in this instance there is a relationship to and one is part of something else such as nature or animal fellowship. Involuntary loneliness on the other hand involves a lack of context and connectedness. To be involuntarily lonely and not belonging to anyone is to lack participation in the world. To not be. Loneliness as a phenomenon is further characterized as transcending the present situation containing loneliness. One can feel lonely even if there are many people around, or one can be completely alone without feeling lonely. Loneliness can disappear with a sense of belonging, when one connects with someone who is miles away.

(p. 195)

We recommend that readers considering using a phenomenological approach in their research, because the research question requires it, take some time to familiarise themselves with the debates within phenomenological research about descriptive and interpretive approaches and to consider a nuanced rationale for their specific phenomenological approach informed by the research question rather than prematurely lurching into 'one camp or the other.' There are many complex considerations, many continuities between approaches, in addition to discontinuities, that rest on a long and deep philosophical heritage and to ignore this complexity and exclusively focus entirely on discontinuities can potentially undermine phenomenology's concerns to offer an alternative epistemology in health care fields. If the study claims to be phenomenological then it needs to reflect what phenomenology is. This does not mean that novice researchers are necessarily required to read continental philosophy *extensively* from the very beginning, although it can be very helpful to do so, but rather they should read some philosophy and find a foundation for what they are choosing to do, and then further deepen and build on their reading drawing on philosophy as they become more expert. There are many philosophical scholars who can act as guides within this arena and whom provide directions that take account of substantial philosophical analyses to underpin credible phenomenological research. In disciplines such as nursing, psychology and education we can be attentive to this 'already digested' informative fundamental philosophical work to guide applications of phenomenology and to also make the most of the extensive methodological literature that has been developing in a range of disciplines. There are also methods texts that consider a variety of schools of phenomenology and which draws distinctions (See, for example, Finlay, 2011). This includes making use of long-established philosophical ideas to further develop insights and generalisations from our findings (Lindberg, Almerud Osterberg, & Horberg, 2016). A further example of this is how the lifeworld constituents (temporality, intersubjectivity, embodiment, spatiality and mood articulated by Husserl, Heidegger, Merleau-Ponty and Medard Boss) can act as guiding dimensions to deepen philosophical analyses and support expression of a general structure with its various constituents through phenomenological reflection sensitised by ideas from philosophy: Todres and Galvin (2010) have done this to delineate dimensions of well-being and also dignity (Galvin & Todres, 2015). A further example is provided by Ashworth concerning lifeworld constituents always implicated in lifeworld experience and can deepen insights from findings, such as sociality, self-hood, embodiment, temporality, discourse, project and moodedness (Ashworth, 2016).

Research process in phenomenological research

As with every research methodology, the applied phenomenological method is a systematic process that includes stages that are interdependent of each other (Englander, 2012; Kvale, 1996). First of all, one has to delineate the phenomenon of interest. As expressed in the examples from health professions provided earlier in this present chapter, descriptive phenomenological research projects seek to understand the general structures of an experience. Take Vuoskoski's (2014) descriptive study on student experience of work-placement assessment. The study itself sought to understand the experience of the experience, placing considerable value on the student's subjective understanding of their work-placement rather than a study on an evaluation of the work-placement If seeking structure and guidance, Giorgi's (2009) method is one example of a step-by-step process which aims to meet scientific criteria of analysis. In summary, the method is based on (1) obtaining and transcribing a raw description of a phenomenon while employing phenomenological reduction, (2) reading for a sense of whole that is situated in the description, (3) maintaining the attitude of the phenomenological reduction, (4) delineating meaning units within the descriptions, (5) highlighting key constituents of the meaning units while using free imaginative variation to 'stress test' the entity of the structure and (6) produce an essential description of the phenomenon through the meaning units (Giorgi et al., 2017). Giorgi (2009) does explain that the whole process must be discipline specific. For example, Giorgi (2009, p. 191) states that a psychologist engaging in the phenomenological method "has to come up with psychological meaning of the details, which is a type of invariance that is different from the philosophical essence".

The interview is considered to be one of the primary procedures used when engaging in phenomenological based research. The purpose of the phenomenological interview is to gather as much detailed descriptions and examples of aspects of the phenomenon under study as possible. Often the interviewer will begin with a very general question, for example, just has to ask "can you tell me about your experience of…" This can then be followed up very simply with for example "Can you share with me any more examples of that…" or "Can you say more about what that was like…" We refer readers to specialist texts to explore more detail regarding phenomenological approaches to interviews in Kvale, 1996; Finlay, 2011 and Wertz et al., 2011. If, however, a researcher seeks to explore phenomenon from the stance of an interpretive phenomenologist, it is not uncommon to employ the use of a semi-structured interview guide that meets a set agenda of interest (Pietkiewicz & Smith, 2012). The guide, according to Pietkiewicz and Smith (2012), supports the interview by offering a number of related topics to cover throughout.

However, Englander (2012) warns of the dangers associated with using any generic techniques to ascertain the data to fulfil the research question. It is the responsibility of the researcher, therefore, to follow the specific philosophical foundations that fall within the distinctive phenomenological traditions. If not done so, Englander (2012) cautions, a researcher runs the risk of methodological fluidity, whereby the whole process has been influenced by two or three phenomenological stances, rather than one defendable position. In typical phenomenological research, for example, interviewing an individual about their experience of certain phenomena, a researcher would attempt to ask questions that are not leading or directly focussed on providing a specific answer. Rather, it is expected that a researcher would ask questions that require more clarification or description of the previous answers the participants have provided (Englander, 2012). Whether the researcher adopts an interpretive or descriptive emphasis, we argue that it is the coherence of the phenomenological approach that is important and that it includes three phenomenologically distinctive features, starts in the lifeworld and is faithful to lifeworld complexity; makes use of a sensitising reflective analytic method or use of 'the reduction' with an arrival at an essential description with wholes and parts and how they fit together, (what qualitative features define the experience most generally but also making meaningful sense of commonalities and unique details between the experience(s) under study). Some interpretive researchers opt for a *fusion of horizons*. Here hermeneutic phenomenologists are also interested in meaning and significance of an experience but express it as meaning being pointed out in multiple ways with a reliance on insights that are personally sensitised by the researcher and with helpful theories. A single specific description may not be reached, but rather the aim is to offer deep understandings that are unique and idiosyncratic. For examples of interpretive hermeneutic work, see Thackery and Eatough (2015, 2018); Eatough, Smith, and Shaw (2008); and Suddick et al. (2019).

There are also many examples of thematic analysis of qualitative data in the literature with claims that it is phenomenology. This is a problem, as phenomenology must rest on the principles we have described if it is to be faithful to its epistemological foundation and cannot be reduced to generic thematic analyses. Some attempts have been made to helpfully mediate this problem i.e. Sundler et al., (2019) in the methods literature. However we wish to emphasise that the steps outlined in this present chapter and the use of 'bridling', after Dahlberg, to remain open to the phenomenon and to be disciplined within a phenomenological attitude alongside deep reflection, rich description and intuiting meanings is central in our view The complex concepts underpinning phenomenology are needed and cannot be easily dropped.

It is also possible of course to engage in phenomenological enquiry philosophically to reach deep insights without 'data', but by using phenomenological reflection and analysis and engagement with phenomenological theory. Philosophical enquiry can also inform health and social care. Examples include using continental philosophy themes in dialogue with issues of body and mind (Gilbert & Lennon, 2005), issues of well-being (Burwood, 2018), and of embodiment (Leder, 1990) as just a few examples.

In empirically based phenomenology, the data that is collected in phenomenological research is from people who can share examples of experiences they have personally lived through. This concerns much more than mere opinions or views, the emphasis is on concrete examples and descriptions of their own personal experiences. Therefore, sampling strategies are determined by the research question that is being asked, participants who have had a direct experience of the phenomenon of interest regardless of age, gender, ethnicity, and other personal factors dependent on the research question. In this respect, sampling in a phenomenological study is not about the demographic of the participants whom are included, as it is the phenomenon that is of interest (Englander, 2012) and this should guide the sampling strategy Phenomenological researchers sometimes utilise "maximum variation sampling" strategies (Giorgi, 2009; Englander, 2012) in order to understand a shared experience from different contexts (Pitney & Parker, 2009). For example Todres and Galvin (2012) included older people who were fully mobile and who could leave their house, older people who were mobile who could not leave their house, for instance because of transport difficulties, older people who were housebound, and older people with poor mobility who could leave their house to form a maximum variation sample in a phenomenological study of the meaning of mobility.

There is also some debate about the use of the literature in phenomenology. The research question should be informed by what is already known about the topic, by what has already been done in the topic and where the gaps in the literature are. This does not preclude any form of reduction or bracketing in our view. Bracketing and phenomenological openness is not about ignoring any knowledge as if it doesn't exist, rather it is about coming back to the literature with an open mind and questioning assumptions that may be evident in the literature, re- looking again, and then putting that aside and engaging with the phenomenon freshly and naively adopting 'phenomenological attitude' and openness to peoples' concrete experiences, letting any insights emerge directly from a return to experiential matters rather than prematurely shaped and influenced by concepts in the literature. It means a coming 'back to the matters' at hand.

In summary, phenomenology is primarily philosophical, but it can be applied as a research approach and several writers have developed different formulations that are descriptive or interpretive and which have been adapted through a range of human science disciplines to form enquiry methodologies and procedures. From this rich movement various methods of data analysis and analytic methods have been formulated for data analysis. There are very many complex debates within this movement about their phenomenological features and claims to be phenomenology which we can't deal with in this present chapter, readers are referred to the extensive methodological literature in the field and are encouraged to explore the debates and critiques concerning the specific kind of phenomenology they are proposing undertaking. The phenomenological approach, is not however, only procedural, but is a *reflective* process aiming to be illuminative about the whatness of a phenomenon with rich description and to offer new insight *about the meaning of a phenomenon*. This meaning may be conveyed in such a way that readers can resonate with the meanings, relate personally to findings, engage with the phenomenon in imaginative ways and in so doing can create a connection with human qualities to contribute to new understanding. This is one reason why phenomenology has been so useful and widely adopted in disciplines in health and social care. The study of human experience is complicated and is not as straightforward as it might at first seem and phenomenology offers great potential to this field. Some critics have argued that descriptions from a first-person perspective are embedded too much in an insider point of view that is problematic and which cannot fully account for human behaviour. These critics hold that it is not the individual that can best explain as what happens in situations and what can explain behaviours that may be shaped by social, cultural or other forces. These forces can be more appropriately analysed by methods that attend to a third person perspective, for example observational methods. However, phenomenology has its key strength in capturing and expressing the meaning of significant human experiences in a rigorous manner, and these forms of knowledge are important in health and social care, such knowledge can be a resource for ethical sensitivity by offering insights that humanise situations and which can lead caring practices.

Contemporary Directions in Phenomenology

Phenomenology has also been developing innovatively in a range of disciplines in a number of very exciting directions each built on distinctive seminal works which include but are not limited to for instance: dialogical phenomenology (see Halling, Rowe, & Leifer, 2006) neurophenomenology (Varela, 1991; Gallagher et al., 2015) and eco-phenomenology (Brown & Toadvine, 2003). These innovative directions in phenomenology are being taken up in environmental science, heritage studies, architecture, and neuroscience to name a few and provide indication of the value of phenomenology in understanding human life in all its complexity. We would like to end this chapter with an indication of the potential of just one of these contemporary developments for the project of phenomenology that strikes at the heart of a sensibility seeking research approaches that can be faithful to human experience in all its complexity. We use this example as an illustration and indication of how the phenomenological approach continues to evolve, with versatility that can span problematic disciplinary perspectives, overcome superficiality and address highly specific research problems concerning human experience and its invisibility in research terms.

Neurophenomenology

Neurophenomenology is an integrated, promising approach to study and explore consciousness from multiple aspects to aid understanding of what consciousness means to us. It is largely influenced through the philosophical work of Merleau-Ponty, in *The Structure of Behaviour*, he "argued for the mutual illumination among phenomenology of direct lived experience, psychology, and neurophysiology". (Varela et al., 1991, p. 15).

In the 1990s, Varela began pushing phenomenology into new directions by encompassing neuroscience with phenomenology. According to Chalmers and Varela, we have come to the problem of consciousness which seems to be insolvable with standard methods of cognitive science (Chalmers, 1995). Therefore, Varela (1996) explored qualitative research and thought phenomenology may have a place in developing research when studying human experience with consciousness. It is widely agreed that experience derives from a physical basis and that we, as humans, are subjects of experience. However, the question of how these systems are subject to experience is still perplexing in neuroscience (Varela, 1996). As Chalmers states, we will never be able to explain the thoughts and feelings of being a human that interacts with the environment only through explaining information processes and mechanisms (Chalmers, 1995). The phenomenological tradition correctly states that studying an objective phenomena always entails a subjective aspect, even more so when studying the complexity of the human mind (Strle, 2013). Therefore, studying a subjective aspect of consciousness in the way in which the world presents itself to oneself, will allow for a richer understanding of human experience and consciousness using neurophenomenology.

In a further example, Reinerman-Jones et al. (2013) investigated the experiences of awe and wonder in space using a simulated space travel scenario. The study encompassed physiological measurements and combined this with experiential enquiry using phenomenological interviewing to explore and delve more deeply into how humans experience space. This is one example of a study that successfully makes use of both first and third person perspectives of a highly complex experience within one research study.

Several researchers have used and developed neurophenomenology to explore the anticipation of epileptic seizures and the on-going conscious states and brain coherent dynamics during a simple perceptual task (Petitmengin, Navarro, & Le Van Quyen, 2007, Lutz et al., 2002). A promising naturalised phenomenological study investigated the anticipation of epileptic seizures in nine individuals using neuroscientific measurements and phenomenological interviews (Petitmengin et al., 2007). Petitmengin and colleagues (2007) employed a neurophenomenological framework to explore whether neurophenomenology could guide and determine each aspect of method to reveal something new about the experience of anticipation of epileptic seizure. They identified from previous studies that the measures used are difficult to interpret, and that there is difficulty understanding correlation between behavioural measures and physiological measures. They conducted two sets of phenomenological interviews for each individual to extract rich descriptions of previous seizures experiences. Corresponding with current literature, less than five minutes prior a seizure onset, EEG readings portrayed a decrease in synchronization neural populations surrounding the epileptic focus in the brain of their sample (Le Van Quyen, Martinerie, Navarro, Boon et al., 2001; Martinerie et al., 1998). However, interestingly, verbal descriptions pointed to a state of fragility several hours before seizure onset suggesting a subjective state of experience evident considerably earlier than these objective readings. This work identifies that individual response does not correspond to the cerebral activity recorded suggesting that the awareness of the pre-reflective experience is central. Additionally, it illustrates enrichment in taking the lived experiences within neurological analysis which can draw together a deeper relationship between the individual and how the world is manifest to them.

Concluding remarks

Husserl's contribution and the contributions of the philosophers that followed him have been important for a whole generation of social theorists, including existential, critical, hermeneutic, feminist and postmodern scholars. Phenomenology has been developing for over a century and it is continuing to evolve in interesting and new ways. At its heart phenomenology seeks to return us back to phenomena for new insight so that we can understand phenomena more fully and deeply. This is not only accounts of individual experiences but also includes appreciation of common themes, universal features and qualities, shared and individual characteristics. The variations uncovered help make sense of the meaning of common foundational or fundamental aspects of experience and we argue is a powerful mediation to superficial analysis of qualitative data, lurches to subjectivism, or over emphasised abstractions and theorisations about human experience. Phenomenology lends itself to a focus on everyday experience and its deep lifeworld heritage makes phenomenology an important and valued approach in the health sciences. Understandings of the complexities of human life with all its vicissitudes is essential if health care is to be led by evidence that takes account of and can be faithful to everyday experience. This kind of knowledge is essential in health and social care, and phenomenology offers an essential epistemology in this regard.

References

Ashworth, P.D. (2016). The lifeworld–enriching qualitative evidence. *Qualitative Research in Psychology*, 13(1), 20–32.

Broome, R.E. (2011). *The phenomenological psychology of police deadly force* (Unpublished doctoral dissertation). Saybrook University, Pasadena, CA, USA.

Brown, C.S., & Toadvine, T. (eds.) (2003). *Eco–phenomenology: Back to the Earth itself.* State University of New York Press: Albany.

Burwood, S. (2018). The existential situation of the patient: Well-being and absence. In K. T. Galvin (Ed.), *Routledge Handbook of Well-being*. Abingdon: Routledge, pp. 133–140.

Chalmers, D.J. (1995). Facing up to the problem of consciousness. *Journal of Consciousness Studies*, 2(3), 200–219.

Dahlberg, H., & Dahlberg, K. (2003). To not make definite what is indefinite. *The Humanistic Psychologist*, 31(4), 34–50. doi:10.1080/c8873267.2003.9986933

Dahlberg, K., Dahlberg, H., & Nystrom, M. (2008). *Reflective lifeworld research* (2nd ed.). Lund, Sweden: Studentlitteteur.

Dahlberg, K. (2007). The enigmatic phenomenon of loneliness. *International Journal of Qualitative Studies on Health and Well-being*, 2(4), 195–207.

Dahlberg, K. (2009). The essence of essences: The search for meaning structures in phenomenological analysis of lifeworld phenomenology. *International Journal of Qualitative Studies on Health and Well-being*, 1(1). doi:10.108011748262050047840S

Eatough, V., Smith, J.A., & Shaw, R. (2008). Women, anger and aggression: An interpretative phenomenological analysis. *Journal of Interpersonal Violence*, 23, 1767–1799.

Englander, M. (2012). The interview: Data collection in descriptive phenomenological human scientific research. *Journal of Phenomenological Psychology*, 43(1), 13–35.

Finlay, L. (2011). *Phenomenology for therapists: Researching the lived world*. London: John Wiley & Sons.

Fitzpatrick, N., & Finlay, L. (2008). 'Frustrating disability': The lived experience of coping with the rehabilitation phase following flexor tendon surgery. *International Journal of Qualitative Studies on Health and Well-being*, 3, 143–154.

Gallagher, S., Reinerman, L., Jonz, B., Bockelman, P., & Trempler, J. (2015). *A neurophenomenology of awe and wonder: Towards a non-reductionist cognitive science*. Basingstoke: Palgrave Macmillan.

Gilbert, P. , & Lennon, K. (2005). *The world, the flesh and the subject: Continental themes in philosophy of mind and body*. Edinburgh: Edinburgh University Press.

Giorgi, A. (2009). *The descriptive phenomenological method in psychology*. Pittsburgh, PA: Duquesne University Press.

Giorgi, A., Giorgi, B., & Morley, J. (2017). The descriptive phenomenological psychological method. In C. Willig & W.S. Rogers (Eds.), *The SAGE handbook of qualitative research in psychology* (2nd ed.), pp. 176–192.

Halling, S., Rowe, J.O., & Leifer, M. (2006). The emergence of the dialogical approach: Forgiving another. In C.T. Fischer (Ed.), *Qualitative research methods for psychologists: Introduction through empirical studies*. New York: Academic Press, pp. 173–212.

Holloway, I., & Todres, L. (2005). The status of method: flexibility, consistency and coherence. In I. Holloway (Ed.), *Qualitative research in health care*. Maidenhead, UK: Routledge, pp. 90–103.

Johansson, K., Ekeberg, M., & Dahlberg, K. (2009) A lifeworld phenomenological study of the experience of falling ill with diabetes. *International Journal of Nursing Studies*, 46(2) 197–203.

Kvale, S. (1996). *InterViews: An introduction to qualitative research interviewing*. Thousand Oaks, CA: SAGE.

Leder, D. (1990). *The absent body*. Chicago, IL: University of Chicago Press.

Le Van Quyen, M., Martinerie, J., Navarro, V., Boon, P., D'Havé, M., Adam, C. et al (2001). Anticipation of epileptic seizures from standard EEG recordings. The Lancet, 357, 183–188.

Lindberg, E., Almerud Osterberg, S., & Horberg, U. (2016). Methodological support for the further abstraction of and philosophical examination of empirical findings in the context of caring science. *International Journal of Qualitative Studies on Health and Well-being*, 11, 1748–2631. doi:10.3402/qhw.v11.30482

Lutz, A., Lachaux, J.-P., Martinerie, J., & Varela, F.J. (2002). Guiding the study of brain dynamics by using first-person data: Synchrony patterns correlate with ongoing conscious states during a simple visual task. *Proceedings of the National Academy of Sciences*, 99(3), 1586–1591. https://doi.org/10.1073/pnas.032658199

Martinerie, J., Adam, C., Le Van Quyen, M., Baulac, M., Clémenceau, S., Renault, B., et al. (1998). Epileptic seizures can be anticipated by non-linear analysis. Nature Medicine, 4:10, 1173–1176.

Moran, D. (2000). *Introduction to phenomenology*. London: Routledge.

Norlyk, A., & Martinsen, B. (2013). The extended arm of health professionals? Relatives' experiences of patient's recovery in a fast-track programme. *Journal of Advanced Nursing*, 69 (8), 1737–1746.

Petitmengin, C., Navarro, V., & Le Van Quyen, M. (2007). Anticipating seizure: Pre-reflective experience at the center of neuro-phenomenology. *Consciousness and Cognition*, 16(3), 746–764. https://doi.org/10.1016/j.concog.2007.05.006

Pietkiewicz, I. & Smith, J.A. (2012) Praktyczny przewodnik interpretacyjnej analizy fenomenologicznej w badaniach jakościowych w psychologii. Czasopismo Psychologiczne, 18(2), 361–369.

Pitney, W.A., & Parker, J. (2009). *Qualitative research in physical activity and the health professions*. Champaign, IL: Human Kinetics, pp. 63–65.

Reinerman-Jones, L., Sollins, B., Gallagher, S., & Janz, B. (2013). Neurophenomenology: An integrated approach to exploring awe and wonder. *South African Journal of Philosophy*. https://doi.org/10.1080/02580136.2013.867397

Saevi, T., & Fornan, A. (2014). Seeing pedagogically, telling phenomenologically - addressing the profound complexity of education. *Phenomenology & Practice*, 6(2), 50–64.

Strle, T. (2013). Why should we study experience more systematically? *Neurophenomenology and Modern Cognitive Science*, 11(4), 376–390. https://doi.org/10.7906/indecs.11.4.3

Spiegelberg, H. (1994). *The phenomenological movement – A historical introduction*. Netherlands: Kluwer Academic.

Suddick, K.M., Cross, V., Vuoskoski, P., Stew, G., & Galvin, K.T. (2019). The acute stroke unit as a meaningful space: The lived experience of health care practitioners. *Health and Place*, 57, 12–21.

Sundler, A. J., Lindberg, E., Nilsson, C., & Palmér, L. (2019). Qualitative thematic analysis based on descriptive phenomenology. *Nursing Open*. 2019;00:1–7.

Thackeray, L., & Eatough, V. (2015). 'Well, the future, that is difficult': A hermeneutic phenomenological analysis exploring the maternal experience of parenting a young adult with a developmental disability. *Journal of Applied Research in Intellectual Disabilities*, 28(4), 265–275.

Thackeray, L., & Eatough, V. (2018) 'Shutting the world out': An interpretative phenomenological analysis exploring the paternal experience of parenting a young adult with a developmental disability. *Journal of Applied Research in Intellectual Disabilities*, 31(S2), 179–190.

Todres, L. (2005). Clarifying the life-world: Descriptive phenomenology. In I. Holloway (Ed.), *Qualitative Research in Health Care*. Maidenhead, UK: Open University Press, pp. 104–124.

Todres, L., & Galvin, K. (2010). 'Dwelling-mobility': An existential theory of well-being. *International Journal of Qualitative Studies on Health and Well-being*, 5(3). doi:10.3402/qhw.v5i3.5444

Todres, L., & Holloway, I. (2004). Descriptive phenomenology: Life-world as evidence. In F. Rapport (Ed.), *New Qualitative Methodologies in Health and Social Care Research*. London: Taylor & Francis, pp. 79–98.

Galvin, K., & Todres, L. (2015). Dignity as honour-hound: An experiential and relational view. *Journal of Evaluation in Clinical Practice*, 21(3),410–418. doi:10.1111/jep.12278

Todres, L., & Galvin, K. (2012). In the middle of everywhere: A phenomenological study of mobility and dwelling amongst rural elders. *Phenomenology and Practice*, 6(1), 55–68.

Varela, F.J. (1996). Neurophenomenology: A methodological remedy for the hard problem. *Journal of Consciousness Studies*, 3(4), 330–349.

Vuoskoski, P. (2014). *Work-placement assessment as a lived-through educationally meaningful experience of the student: An application of the phenomenological descriptive approach* (Unpublished doctoral thesis). University of Jyväskylä, Finland.

Wertz, F.J., Charmaz, K., Mc Mullen, L.M., Josselon, R., AndersonR., & McSpadden, E. (2011). *Five ways of doing qualitative analysis*. New York: Guildford Press.

Zahavi, D. (2019). *Phenomenology: The basics*. New York: Routledge.

7

PHENOMENOLOGY – QUESTIONING CONSCIOUSNESS AND EXPERIENCE

Graham Stew

Introduction

Right now, as you read these words on this page, you are presumably having a conscious experience. If you stop and ask yourself: "Am I conscious now?" the answer will naturally be 'Yes'. But how do you know? ... and what does being conscious mean? If we are honest, we cannot even begin to understand consciousness. It is the most obvious and intimate of things, but philosophers and scientists have failed to produce any convincing explanations, and it remains a total mystery.

> "There is nothing we know more intimately than conscious experience, but there is nothing that is harder to explain."
>
> *—David Chalmers, 1995a, p. 200*

Is it possible for the eye to see itself . . . or to know that which is knowing? The conclusion is that the subject of consciousness always eludes us, as it is its own object.

Social researchers, and in particular, phenomenologists, seek to understand the inner world of our feelings, attitudes, sensations, and the meanings we attach to our experience. The resulting research ends up describing and interpreting (sometimes even explaining) our subjective experience and behaviour, without considering the origin of these phenomena. It is like being fascinated by the images on a TV screen, whilst ignoring the electricity and broadcasting system which produce them.

This chapter sets out to explore consciousness and experience, the fundamental aspects of being human. Using phenomenology (the study of the phenomenal) as our focus, we shall address the noumenal, that which is the source of all

126 Graham Stew

appearances. Western science and eastern philosophy will be visited in our search, and a range of theories, both materialist and metaphysical, will be discussed. Rather than situating my discussion within a humanist <->post-humanist dimension, much of what will be covered could be seen as 'post-theoretical', as it transcends current categories of discourse. In so doing I shall be challenging our Eurocentric views of consciousness, awareness and experience. The implications for phenomenological researchers will be considered in a final section.

Phenomenology

Phenomenology is defined as the study of the objects of consciousness, as they appear to individual awareness. From the Greek *phainomenon*, meaning appearance, phenomena are the sensations, thoughts and perceptions which constitute the totality of our lived experience. The emphasis of phenomenology is on the world as lived by individuals (their 'life-world'), not the world or reality as something separate from subjective experience. This approach to research asks "What is this experience like?" as it attempts to explore meanings as they are lived in everyday life.

Phenomenology as a branch of philosophy has a long history originating in the work of Plato and his distinction between sensory and abstract experiences. The themes of phenomenology were explored by Kant, Schopenhauer, Berkeley and Hume, but became prominent at the end of the 19th century as a result of the work of Franz Brentano (1973) and William James (1890). The inner subjective world, capable of exploration through introspection, became a focus of interest as a reaction against the objective materialism of science.

The founding figure of phenomenology, Edmund Husserl (1859–1938), sought to establish an equally rigorous science of subjective experience. The intention was to investigate methodically the essential structures of consciousness, whilst adopting the 'phenomenological attitude', where prior understanding and knowledge were deliberately suspended; the so-called 'bracketing' or *epoché*. This suspension of the 'natural' pre-reflective attitude was intended to open the researcher's mind to broader possibilities of meaning. Objects of consciousness could therefore be described in terms of their essential and invariant features; those characteristics of a phenomenon without which it could not be regarded as such.

An epistemological emphasis was evident in the desire to formulate objective accounts of subjective phenomena, e.g. the experiences of loneliness or of becoming a parent. The emphasis is on the reduction of associations and meanings to a specific and pure description of such experiences, in order to increase our understanding and establish a science of consciousness. In not denying the existence of an external world, it could be argued that Husserl inadvertently re-instated the subject–object division that was then regarded as the flaw in logical positivism.

Later phenomenologists, such as Martin Heidegger (1889–1976), developed a more ontological focus, with an interest in interpreting the socio-cultural and historical context of experience. There was an acceptance of researchers' pre-understandings as a necessary and inevitable component of any inquiry, and any attempt at 'bracketing' prior assumptions was abandoned. For Heidegger, to be human is to be an interpreter of experience, and all understanding is an act of interpretation.

All phenomenologists claim to explore 'lived experience' and the phenomena that appear to consciousness. However, there are differences in the emphasis of this process, in that researchers will either attempt to describe or interpret individuals' experience. They can ask: "What is this experience like?" or "What is it like to be a person living with this experience/disease?" There is a clear shift between an epistemological (knowing) and an ontological (being) focus – a subtle but significant distinction. Either there is a reductive focus on essential features of an experience, or an inclusive acceptance of contextual factors; either a bracketing out of prior understanding, or a mutual co-construction of meaning between researcher and participant.

This chapter is not concerned with the internecine arguments between phenomenologists, and so the detailed differences between the various schools of thought will not be discussed in depth here. Some aspects of both descriptive and interpretive approaches will be revisited later where appropriate. To summarise, phenomenology is concerned with understanding the meaning, impact and significance of experience for individuals. It does not claim generalisability and does not seek to generate theory. Instead phenomenologists argue that achieving deep and meaningful insights into how individuals perceive their experience (e.g. pain) will provide for more sensitive and aware responses (e.g. in health professionals).

Phenomenology as a research methodology is not well charted, as phenomenological philosophers tended not to undertake research, and left no models or 'recipes' for investigating conscious experience. We do, however, have some guidance from recent writers such as Giorgi (2009) as a descriptive phenomenologist, and Smith, Flowers, and Larkin (2009), who employ an interpretive approach in interpretative phenomenological analysis. We also have earnest debates over just what constitutes phenomenology (e.g. van Manen, 2017), and whether hermeneutics can be regarded as having a role within phenomenology. Other phenomenologists such as Merleau-Ponty and Gadamer have stressed the embodied nature of experience and the importance of language. Researchers therefore need to reflect on the fundamental purpose of their inquiries and adopt a methodology consistent with these aims.

What seems to be missing from much current debate is the nature of our inner subjective world. Just what is consciousness and what do we mean when we talk about experience? The following sections of the chapter will take phenomenology's central focus of consciousness and experience and explore what these concepts might mean. No conclusive answers will be revealed, as these matters remain a mystery to both philosophers and scientists. However, some general remarks on the implications for today's researchers, and a few more questions, will be discussed at the end.

128 Graham Stew

What is consciousness?

Ask yourself again: "Am I conscious now?" If the answer is Yes . . . what are you conscious of? Phenomenologists will assert that we are always conscious *of* something, be it a thought, sensation or emotion. Whatever becomes the focus of our attention is an object of consciousness, an act of reference. This direction of attention toward a phenomenon appearing in consciousness was termed *'intentionality'* by Franz Brentano (1838–1917). Thus, we are always conscious or aware of or about something, and Husserl's phenomenology was based on this intentionality of consciousness. Not only is consciousness always directed towards an object, but every conscious experience exists as a *noema*. Husserl used this term to represent the object or content of a thought, judgement, or perception, but scholars are still unsure of its precise meaning in his work. *Noesis* is the apprehension or intellectual reasoning which perceives the object of consciousness (the noema).

Husserl (1980) also described pure foundational consciousness as a transcendental subjectivity which is achieved through the phenomenological reduction known as *epoché*. As previously described, this is the deliberate identification and suspension of the so-called pre-reflective or 'natural' attitude. This attitude consists of our prior understanding, assumptions and all theoretical knowledge related to the object in question. Through this 'bracketing' of fore-structures of understanding Husserl argued that the pure and essential structures of an experience can be revealed and described. In this sense he could be regarded as an idealist, asserting that subjective experience was the ground of absolute existence and that an apparent external world consisted only of consciousness (Puligandla, 1970)

But let us return to our central question ... what does it mean to be conscious? We perceive an unconscious 'material' world and wonder where consciousness comes from. I am using the term 'consciousness' in this chapter to mean all the sensory and mental events of awareness. These include the sensations of colours, shapes, sounds, tastes, smells and touch, and all mental thoughts, feelings, memories and images. Thus, I am referring to the phenomenon of being conscious, rather than to the neurological processes that make these subjective experiences possible.

Right now I am conscious of a Mozart symphony. I know that sound waves are reaching my ears and being converted into action potentials which travel along the cochlear nerves to my auditory cortex. What happens to transform these electrical and chemical activities into the subjective experience of beautiful music? How can a few pounds of grey, wet tissue create the smell of coffee, the taste of a peach, and even images of non-existent objects such as centaurs or unicorns? Why should several billion interacting neurones give rise to a subjective sense of presence . . . of simply being here?

This is the 'hard problem' famously defined by David Chalmers:

> *"The hard problem is the question of how physical processes in the brain give rise to subjective experience." –Chalmers, 1995b, p. 63*

Phenomenology – questioning consciousness **129**

The 'easy' problems of consciousness have been tackled over the last century and include cognition, attention, sleep, behaviour, and memory. Functional MRI scans have told us much about neural activity within the brain, but the 'explanatory gap' between the objective material brain and the subjective world of experience remains unbridgeable. Some neuroscientists insist that once all the easy problems have been solved, the hard problem will disappear. Others are not so optimistic; suggesting that there is no way that science can explain consciousness, because consciousness *is* what knows science (Wallace, 2000). Let us look at some of the theories that have been proposed to explain the mystery of consciousness, or as Alan Watts (2017) put it: to 'eff' the ineffable.

Philosophical and psychological theories of consciousness

The first recorded accounts of human consciousness can be found in the Indian Upanishads and other Vedic scriptures, dating back to the sixth century BCE, and predating the Greek philosophers who laid the foundations for western philosophy. I shall be touching on the non-dual viewpoint of Advaita Vedanta later, but basically consciousness here is seen as the source of all experience, and that all experience appears within conscious awareness. Existence and awareness of existence are inseparable. Non-dual awareness contains subject and object, and there are no external physical objects.

Indian and Buddhist philosophy view self-luminous consciousness as revealing itself *to itself*. There is no self or ego separate from consciousness, but the story of the self is constructed through the conditioned interpretation of experience. Buddhism thus denies the existence of a persisting self, which is simply viewed as a series of transient perceptions giving the illusion of continuity.

A contemporary philosopher and consciousness researcher, K. Ramakrishna Rao (2011)states:

> Consciousness in the Indian tradition is more than an experience of awareness. It is a fundamental principle which underlies all knowing and being . . . the cognitive structure does not generate consciousness; it simply reflects it; and in the process limits and embellishes it. In a fundamental sense, consciousness is the source of our awareness. In other words, consciousness is not merely awareness as manifest in different forms but it is also what makes awareness possible. . . . It is the light which illuminates the things on which it shines.
>
> *(p. 335)*

Materialism and idealism

We now come to the debates between materialists and idealists, and between dualists and monists. The arguments are complex and often hidden behind obscure and difficult concepts, so I shall attempt to keep things simple.

Monists argue that there is only one kind of stuff in the universe . . . whilst dualists claim that there are two kinds of stuff. Perhaps the best known dualist theory is that of René Descartes (1596–1650), who theorised that there are two realms of existence, the physical and the non-physical spirit or soul (Cartesian dualism). He proposed that the brain and the mind were made of different substances; that the brain and body were physical and made of matter, whilst the mind and all mental activity were non-physical. The problem with this proposal is evident … how do the two interact? Descartes suggested that they met at the pineal gland, situated in the centre of the brain, but provided no explanation of how the physical realm communicates with the mental. As Susan Blackmore (2005) points out,

> This problem of interaction bedevils any attempt to build a dualist theory, which is probably why most philosophers and scientists completely reject all forms of dualism in favour of some kind of monism; but the options are few and also problematic.
>
> *(p. 4)*

Monist theorists argue that either the mental world is foundational (idealism), or that all things consist of matter (materialism). A century after Descartes, the philosopher George Berkeley (1685–1753) claimed that all experience of the world arises from mental perception. Samuel Johnson famously rejected this theory by kicking a large stone and asserting, "I refute it *thus*!" This action merely dismissed Berkeley's argument, rather than proving the existence of the stone was independent of its perception.

Idealism and monism have a long history as Indian and Buddhist thought embrace this perspective. Here the world and all objects are viewed as the products of consciousness and mental activity, and the idea of an external and independent world is rejected. Consciousness is the primary reality, the physical world being ultimately illusory (Watts, 1976; Loy, 1988; Waite, 2007; Timalsina, 2009).

Materialism is a monist position and maintains that primary reality is physical, the mind being the physical and functional properties of the brain and having a scientific explanation. Consciousness has a physical basis and is an *epiphenomenon* in that it derives from brain activity. An objective world exists independently of the observer. This reductive materialism remains the dominant paradigm for the world's scientific community and positivist research generally. Neuroscientists are seeking the neural correlates of consciousness and believe they will ultimately identify the physical source of mental experience. The frustrating anomaly for the current paradigm is consciousness itself; it cannot be doubted and yet it cannot be explained.

Our everyday experience suggests that somewhere inside our heads is a small person who is watching the outside world, making decisions and controlling our actions. This 'I' is sitting in what Daniel Dennett (1991) has termed a "Cartesian theatre", and here we experience sensations, thoughts and feelings; the whole 'show' of life as a stream of consciousness. Dennett rejects this notion, as the brain simply does not work this way. Information is received by different centres and is distributed for purposes to many areas of the cerebral cortex. There is (as yet) no known place or process in the brain that could be responsible for producing conscious experience. There is no way in which all sensory input can be brought together in one 'seat of consciousness', and there is no little person to experience and act upon the unfolding appearances. So perhaps the theatre has no audience, and we are participants rather than spectators?

The tool we use for wrestling with these questions is the human mind. A major challenge is that we cannot be certain anything exists outside the mind, because the mind is the main agent for exploring this question. Apparently, there is a German word that captures the problem: *unhintergehbarkeit*. The nearest translation is something like: 'ungetbehindability'. We are stuck with our minds (which appear in consciousness), and there seems no way to get behind them. Until they fall silent . . . and then maybe . . . ?

The development of psychology

William James (1842–1910), the father of modern psychology, advocated introspection to study the stream of consciousness; the continuous flow of sensations, images, thoughts and feelings that we experience. His approach was predominantly monist in that he rejected dualist concepts and placed consciousness at the heart of his psychology, viewed as the science of mental life. Introspection had been initially developed by Wilhelm Wundt (1897) and Edward Titchener (1901) who were keen to make systematic and reliable observations of inner experiences such as attention and sensation.

This interest in the inner life was developed further by Sigmund Freud (1915/2000) with his theories of the unconscious and psychoanalysis. Elsewhere in Europe the emerging concepts of existentialism and phenomenology were regarded as significant. As we have seen, Husserl's (1970) seminal work in phenomenology sought to 'get back to the things themselves', and develop a systematic approach to investigating conscious experience. This interest in establishing a transcendental science of consciousness is challenged by its very subjectivity: how can one decide between conflicting claims for private experience?

These problems led to the study of introspection being superseded by a movement in psychology which dominated most of the twentieth century - behaviourism. Behaviourists such as John B. Watson (1924) and B.F. Skinner (1953) dismissed introspection and consciousness as irrelevant to the objective and measurable science of psychology, whose goal was the prediction and control of human behaviour. The dominant paradigm of scientific materialism has regarded subjectivity as something of a taboo (Wallace, 2000), and this view has restricted systematic inquiry into the nature and potential of consciousness.

The dominance of behaviourism continued until the 1980s. Mental states and attitudes, problem solving and cognitive processing were all investigated, but no true introspection into one's inner life (as advocated by James) was undertaken seriously. The current metaparadigm of western science still asserts that the real

132 Graham Stew

world is the material world, and that space, time, and energy are primarily by-products of insentient matter.

This unquestioned assumption of materialism, and other theories, were explored and challenged in the 1980s and 90s by a wide range of writers who have revived the science of consciousness (Baars, 1988; Dennett, 1991; Penrose, 1995; Crick, 1994; Lycan, 1996; Chalmers, 1996). The new interest in the nature of consciousness has also resulted in a proliferation of published research and related journals (e.g. *The Journal of Consciousness Studies, Consciousness and Cognition, Psyche*), and also the creation of professional societies and conferences, e.g. the Association for the Scientific Study of Consciousness (ASSC).

Yet still: "Human consciousness is just about the last surviving mystery" (Dennett, 1991, p. 21). Centuries of philosophical and scientific inquiry have not produced any means by which consciousness can be detected, and we do not know what exactly is to be measured. As Wallace (2000) points out, at present there is no scientific evidence even for the existence of consciousness. We only have our own first-person accounts of what it means to be conscious.

We understand a great deal about perception, visual attention, reactions to stimuli, and various cognitive and behavioural functions. But why are they accompanied by subjective experience? Why should all these physical processes produce this sense of presence . . . this background hum of being . . . this inner life?

There may be no bigger question, but western philosophers and scientists don't have a clue what any answer would look like. For all its successes in explaining the working of the universe and improving human life, science has failed conspicuously to provide any convincing explanation of the very thing that conceived it – consciousness itself. As the famous astrophysicist Sir Arthur Eddington (1928) said: "Something unknown is doing we don't know what!"

What is experience?

Phenomenology seeks to understand "lived experience", but what does that really mean? Put simply, our experience consists of sensations, thoughts and feelings which result from sensory perceptions and mental activity.

Simple perceptions such as the taste of an orange, the smell of coffee, or the colour blue are known to philosophers as *qualia* (Blackmore, 2005). These building blocks of experience might be regarded as the raw 'givens' of perception prior to interpretation. Are these the essential structures that phenomenologists seek . . . the 'things themselves'? Do we see, hear, taste, touch and smell objects as they appear *in* consciousness . . . or *as* consciousness? If they are regarded as 'external' objects, there is an assumption of a subject who is experiencing them in time and space. This is the conventional view of human sentience . . . the first-person account of our inner experience. But how does it stand up to critical examination?

What can be said about mental phenomena such as thoughts, emotions, memories, ideas and images? They appear in awareness, spontaneously and uninvited, but we usually claim ownership and responsibility for them (*my* thoughts, feelings, etc.). Descriptive phenomenologists aim to capture the 'pre-reflective' nature of our experience, before the layers of thoughts, theory and judgment obscure our perception. Can these be immaculate perceptions; a form of choiceless awareness before the movement of thought? Many contemplative traditions (in both the East and West) would contend that it is possible to reach such an open and empty state of receptivity (Krishnamurti, 2010). Indeed they would question the assumption of an 'experiencer' who experiences . . . a subject who perceives objects. We will visit this perspective later in the chapter.

So, let us now recap. Experience comprises mental events and sensory information which seems to produce an inner world of subjective experience . . . of being. Upon further investigation it can be argued that the concepts of time and space, and indeed of a separate self, are also produced by the interpreted construction of experience. The world and our assumed identity are understood and conceptualised through this ever-changing flow of phenomena . . . the 'stream of consciousness' first described by William James (1890).

All experience requires conscious awareness in order to be experienced. Mind, which appears in consciousness, is necessary for the world to exist. Quantum physicists are recognising the fundamental nature of consciousness, viewing the universe as a 'self-excited circuit' which gives rise to consciousness, which in turn gives meaning to the universe (see Bohm, 1980; Herbert, 1985; Tiller, 1997; Capra, 2010). Quantum theory cannot be completely defined without introducing features of consciousness. This view of the primacy of consciousness is gathering increasing support in the scientific community and seems likely to sweep away the obsolete but still dominant paradigm of reductive materialism.

In this new paradigm consciousness is fundamental. It enables experience to create meaning and understanding, and it is the one thing we cannot deny. *(Are you still conscious? If you are reading these words, of course you are!)* So, experiences appear in consciousness (which is outside time and space, without any characteristics and not locatable) and assume the being-ness of presence. There are no separate phenomena but simply appearances in and *as* consciousness. Objects exist in the abstract world of thought and are concepts rather than actual entities.

Is there an enduring self or ego that is aware of experience? As already discussed, experience can be regarded as a series of interconnected events and mental states (thoughts, feelings and sensations). The assumption of the continued existence of an ego (or subject who experiences) is challenged not only by Buddhist thought, but other theorists, such as Derek Parfit (1986) and his 'bundle' theory of self. Drawing upon the ideas of David Hume (1711–1776), Parfit claims that all experiences and mental events are causally related and can be likened to a 'bundle' tied up with string. One can examine experiences seeking for a 'self' who experiences, but all that is found are the experiences. What I may regard as 'my life' is a series of perceptions and impressions which are tied together by memory and give rise to the idea of an enduring identity. There is no person apart from the series of connected events, and what we call an individual is merely a convention of language.

Such a theory seems counter-intuitive, and entails abandoning any belief that you are a person who has free will and lives a life in your particular body. Because of the difficulties in otherwise defining the self, it is a perspective which at least deserves attention. Standing apart from other major religions which support the concept of an ego or soul, Buddhism maintains that there is no substantial or enduring entity that can be regarded as a self, a basic principle (*anatman*) recognised as one of the marks of existence. The Buddha could therefore be viewed as the first bundle theorist. This is not stating that some form of subjectivity does not exist; but that the concept of a persisting and separate self/ego is an illusion . . . it is not what it seems. Viewing the ego as a defined persona or social role, one can see that it consists of an arbitrary selection of experiences with which we have been taught to identify. Why, for example, do we say "I think" but not "I am beating my heart"? (Watts, 2017).

Although denying the ultimate existence of an enduring self, Buddhism admits an impermanent form of subjectivity or sentience . . . the awareness of being present. So, can there can an impersonal awareness, similar to the transcendental consciousness of Husserl (1970) or the 'witness-consciousness' of Advaita Vedanta? Anticipating Husserl, the seventh-century Indian Buddhist thinker Dharmakirti (Dreyfus & Thompson, 2007) argued that conscious states are immanently self-reflexive, and therefore phenomenal. Their 'givenness' provides experiences with their 'seeming' quality; such as how the taste of honey, or the memory of a place, seems 'to be like' something (Nagel, 1974).

We need not assume that a series of experiences requires an independent 'experiencer'. Awareness itself can be regarded as non-dual (having neither subject nor object), and being one with the noumenon, which is the source of all phenomena. It is the movement of thought (which is mind) that disturbs awareness by perceiving, defining and judging apparent objects and states. It follows that, situated within the constructs of time and space, the story of a self can be created.

This sense of self is very real (as 'you' are no doubt aware), and it is this quality of personal subjectivity that makes the whole question of consciousness so puzzling and intriguing. The idea of 'me', with a personal history and identity, is apparently convincing, but to infer that subjective experience proves the existence of a stable, historical person could be a mistake.

The self is a narrative construction as far as Daniel Dennett (1991, p. 246) is concerned: "Our tales are spun, but for the most part we don't spin them; they spin us. Our human consciousness, and our narrative selfhood, is their product, not source." The reification of self is the result of assuming that the transient stream of experience necessarily indicates the existence of a substantive or permanent self or ego.

Can there be a 'subjectivity' of experience . . . the phenomenological focus . . . without reifying a person who is permanent and invariant? There are definite similarities here between Zahavi's (2005) concept of a 'minimal self', the transcendental ego of Husserl, and the witness-consciousness of Vedanta. Could it be this neutral pre-reflective awareness that simply knows the background hum of presence . . . of simply being? Is there a need for an intermediate 'self', which would simply be another phenomenal object?

Buddhism views all objects, including apparent persons, as inherently empty (*shunya*) and impermanent (*anicca*) . . . their existence being illusory. The analogy of a burning candle is often used to explain this position. The light from the candle appears persistent, as the stream of hot flowing gases suggests permanence, but the reality is far from stable and static. Any notion of 'self' is an attempt to capture and halt the flow of life itself . . . there is nothing apart from the appearances . . . nobody is looking on! Mind is needed for the world to exist; and consciousness is necessary for the mind to appear. Consciousness is viewed as the noumenal ground of being by non-dualists as it is self-illuminating and reveals itself by its very occurrence (MacKenzie, 2007).

These ideas may seem challenging for readers who are steeped in familiar Cartesian dualism, and feel comfortable with their realist ontology. However, let me summarise this position as concisely as possible. It is suggested that experience is not produced by the mind but is in consciousness. All experience *is* mind . . . it does not appear in the mind. Mind comprises thoughts, sensations and perceptions, and they all appear in consciousness. All that is experienced is in consciousness and it is consciousness that is experiencing it. There is thinking, feeling and sensing and all these are suffused with consciousness. Consciousness is first-person experience; the knowing element in every experience (Spira, 2017).

We can now move to explore the nature of awareness, but if your brain is hurting too much you may need to take a break!

What is awareness?

If phenomenology is the study of the contents of conscious awareness, who or what is aware?

Does awareness require a self to 'have' awareness? Could it be that at source we are nothing more than conscious awareness? Can consciousness become aware of itself through the appearance of phenomena? Vedantins and Buddhists feel that consciousness is analogous to light, which, in revealing other things, shines in itself (MacKenzie, 2007). Rupert Spira (2017) suggests that awareness knows itself simply by being itself, just as the sun illuminates itself simply by being itself.

Any experience requires the presence of consciousness; but the screen of awareness does not depend on experience. All there is to any experience is sensation and perception. All there is to a sensation or perception is the experience of sensing and perceiving; and the only substance present in sensing and perceiving is awareness.

As nervous systems develop, conditioned by educational and sociocultural influences, apparent objects are recognised from memory and automatically identified when perceived. Familiar objects in the 'developed' world, such as a mobile phone, are instantly labelled; although the same object might mean nothing to a member of a remote Amazonian tribe. Meaning is attached to words and concepts,

136 Graham Stew

and these interpretations are subjective and unique. The mind therefore constructs our 'personal' world, and the mind is made out of consciousness, which is all there is.

This is not solipsism, as it is not suggested that the individual mind is all that can be known to exist. Nor is it pan-psychism, which is still essentially dualistic in viewing everything in the physical world to be imbued with consciousness. We in the West have tended to equate consciousness with subjectivity, which we associate with the mind as a reflection of the body and world. Eastern philosophy, however, distinguishes mind from consciousness, with mind defined as the content of consciousness.

As a sensation or thought is perceived, attention is directed towards it ('intentionality') and the mind (a collection of memories and concepts) is engaged in creating meaning. Attention is simply focussed awareness, which is itself empty and without any qualities. Attention directed outwards towards sensations and thoughts (experience) forms the basis of phenomena (objectification). It is the input from our senses and the resulting mental activity that constitutes our lived experience, and this all occurs within conscious awareness. For any object – a thought, feeling, sensation or perception – to come into the field of experience, consciousness must focus and thus limit its awareness in the form of attention. Attention thus brings form into existence out of the formless field of infinite consciousness. Attention directed inwards to awareness itself (noumenon) is true meditation.

Paying conscious and non-judgmental attention to our moment to moment experience is the essence of mindfulness. Through cultivating this practice, it becomes possible to observe the transient nature of thoughts, feeling and sensations as they arise and pass away in our awareness. Whatever is recognised as an object of one's attention cannot be what one truly is. Mindfulness as a form of conscious and active reflexivity for all researchers probably deserves wider recognition and debate.

Quantum theory has something to contribute to the debate on attention. One of the most significant conclusions reached by quantum physicists in recent times is the fact that no object exists unless it is observed (Schrödinger, 2009; Heisenberg, 2000). There is an interdependent and intimate relationship between the observer and the observed; both are needed for any observation to occur. When there is only observing, the observer becomes the observed (Krishnamurti, 2010). In other words, there is a collapse of both subject and object, from duality to the non-dual; and from the phenomenal to the noumenal.

Applications to the research process

Phenomenological researchers may be reading this chapter and wondering what conclusions to draw from the preceding discussion. Of what relevance are these complex and confusing philosophical ideas to the practical business of doing research?

As phenomenologists we are interested in the experiences and 'lifeworlds' of our participants. Whether our aim is the description of 'essential structures' of a phenomenon of interest, or its interpretation in its existential context, we will hold certain assumptions about the nature of consciousness and experience. These presuppositions may well be unconscious and unquestioned, but the purpose of this chapter has been to bring these issues into the open for critical examination.

Researchers are normally encouraged to make explicit their ontological and epistemological stances, and to explain their philosophical position regarding what constitutes reality and knowledge. In my experience this expectation seems to apply more to qualitative studies than to positivist research.

For phenomenological inquiries, however, there is arguably a need to go further and to consider and justify how the specific approach chosen is consistent with its foundational philosophy.

Certain questions need to be addressed: 'How is consciousness viewed?' 'Does it arise from matter and is a function of the brain?' 'Is there an external, independent world which gives to consciousness?' 'Does experience happen to an individual?' Alternatively: 'Does consciousness give rise to the brain, the world and all phenomena?' 'Does experience create the individual?' 'Can there be description without interpretation?' 'Is the self/ego a construction?' 'Does experience have inherent meaning?' This chapter has not provided any conclusive answers to these questions but has endeavoured to expand the debate on these issues beyond the usual occidental worldview. For example, the Indian concept of witness-consciousness relates to Husserl's transcendental ego and deserves further investigation.

Perhaps in his search for 'pure consciousness' Husserl chose not to venture too far into spiritual traditions, fearing the negative reactions of a positivist world, sceptical of any metaphysics. Would this be seen as a neo-Kantian form of transcendental idealism, too close to 'unknowable spirituality' to be accepted by his conservative academic colleagues? Clinging to forms, he thus developed the empirical and transcendental egos, and the concepts of *noesis* and *noema*: ways of knowing the 'intersubjective natural world-about-me'.

Heidegger sought to move phenomenology to a more existential focus on being-in-the-world (*Dasein*), with a rejection of pure 'mentalism'. He retained the term 'human being' which suggests that he had shifted the earlier consciousness-centred phenomenology to the ontic dimension of anthropology.

Debate continues among philosophers and researchers on the concepts of epoché and reduction, and whether prior understanding, judgements and assumptions can be identified, suspended and transcended, or whether our perceptions are inevitably interpreted and meaning is already present. The subtleties of this debate have not been addressed here, as it has been suggested that phenomena have no inherent or independent existence, dependent as they are on conscious awareness and subject to socio-cultural conditioning. Description always requires interpretation, as we seek to make sense of our experience. Caution is therefore necessary in claiming any type of veracity or wider application for phenomenological findings.

Whichever approach is adopted, the purpose of phenomenology is to gain insight into, and understanding of, individuals' experiences. Awareness, empathy and sensitivity towards a human situation, without claiming generalisability to

138 Graham Stew

wider populations, are regarded as being intrinsically worthwhile and valuable outcomes. In health care settings phenomenological research aims to inform practice and sensitise practitioners. No recommendations or theoretical models are produced as it is up to readers to interpret the findings, and if these resonate with their own experience, the research is likely to have an impact. The researcher's responsibility is to demonstrate reflexivity, authenticity and trustworthiness.

Allow me to propose again that all experience arises within awareness and that the 'reality' we believe we know is actually produced by conceptual thought. We perceive a common world by agreeing on the way we describe it. That is, by labelling objects arising in consciousness, we produce a standardised model of the world using language. Objects and the thoughts that define them seem to arise simultaneously in awareness. We are trapped by language, which is inevitably limited, subjective and dualistic. This mental division of subject and object fractures reality, the true nature of which is non-dual. The belief that objects exist independently of awareness is just that . . . a belief without any foundation of evidence.

To use the familiar metaphor of waves and ocean: the waves (the objects) are the phenomena that we witness with our senses, but their real essence is the ocean (the Subject/Consciousness). The ocean is of course the essence of our true being, but we cannot grasp this with our rational mind. However, when the illusion of being a separate individual is seen through, the identification with the waves disappears and 'ocean-consciousness' comes to the fore. We recognise that both wave and ocean are essentially water, and that everything in the world is interconnected. It is one universal Energy; what Tibetan Buddhists refer to as 'One Taste'.

I am suggesting that being and consciousness are one and the same. There is no such thing as 'objective' being without consciousness; all being is subjective and occurs in and as consciousness. Consciousness is not a 'thing'; it is a capacity to perceive, an openness which is both empty and full. Concepts are objects appearing in awareness, and all experience exists within, and is made of, this conscious awareness. As phenomenology is the study of experience, perhaps it is wise to consider that no 'thing' exists outside consciousness, which is the true nature of our apparent selves and the world. In the light of this understanding, all conceptual debates about description and interpretation pale into insignificance. Husserl's warning is still valid: subjectivity cannot be known by any objective science.

We continue to pay attention to the transitory images on the screen, but not to the screen of awareness itself. It would seem more useful to explore the nature of conscious awareness, without which nothing can be known, or indeed exist. Without an appreciation of the ground of our being, noumenal awareness, there can only be limited understanding of what we call phenomena. As William Blake said, "If the doors of perception were cleansed everything would appear as it is, Infinite" (Carabine, 2000).

Arguably, research will always be a dualistic activity as it sets up a subject to investigate objects. No matter how relativist or constructivist our ontological stance may be, there will inevitably be the division between the researcher and the researched. Whatever theoretical perspective may be adopted . . . existentialism, post-modernism, post-structuralism, post-humanism, or any other 'ism' . . . it will remain simply a conceptual framework through which experiences assume meaning, and which is contained within consciousness. We may make our choice between styles of phenomenology, but need to ensure that our philosophical foundations are sound, defensible and consistent with our aims and outcomes.

We can attempt to restrain prior understanding through consciously adopting a phenomenological attitude, but in reality all experience is one seamless substance. The division between the internal self and the external object is never actually experienced. It is always imagined by thought.

If consciousness is all there is, and all phenomena are simply the contents of consciousness, then what is phenomenological research for? We may explore experience, but any resulting description and interpretation will occur within conscious awareness, which is beyond all analysis and definition. By all means let us study experience, but do not claim it is a science of consciousness, for what will be studied will be doing the studying, and the eye cannot see itself!

Conclusions

So let me summarise and return to phenomenology for the last time. To the researcher asking questions of others about their experience and what it means. To the researcher writing a story about the participants' stories; and the readers of the research taking away their own interpreted stories. What does it all mean?

We explore ... we seek meaning in life ... in our own and others' lives. We do not accept what we find as absolute truth, because we accept that no such thing exists. We understand more; we appreciate others' experiences more deeply, more sensitively . . . and we take those insights into our own lives. These insights may change the way we work and relate to others and ourselves . . . or they may not. Does it matter? Have we increased our store of 'knowledge' as a result of these efforts? Perhaps. Will this knowledge change the world? Probably not.

But human curiosity is indomitable and will not be denied. We ask questions, and demand answers. Phenomenology seeks to satisfy our curiosity about what it means to be human and have experiences. We have little idea what experience is, or where it comes from. We have even less idea about what it means to be conscious, but the thirst for understanding drives us on.

Perhaps we can simply agree that:

The world is known by the senses.
The senses are known by the mind.
The mind is known by Consciousness.
And Consciousness is known by itself.
When we search deep inside Consciousness,
Consciousness searches deep inside us.

140 Graham Stew

References

Baars, B. J. (1988) *A Cognitive Theory of Consciousness*. New York: Cambridge University Press.

Blackmore, S. (2005) *Consciousness: A Very Short Introduction*. Oxford: Oxford University Press.

Bohm, D. (1980) *Wholeness and the Implicate Order*. London: Routledge.

Brentano, F. (1973) *Psychology from an Empirical Standpoint*. London: Routledge. (Original work published 1874).

Capra, F. (2010) *The Tao of Physics: An Exploration of the Parallels Between Modern Physics and Eastern Mysticism* (5th ed.). Boston, MA: Shambhala Publications.

Carabine, K. (ed.) (2000) *The Selected Poems of William Blake* [The Marriage of Heaven and Hell]. London: Wordsworth Editions, pp. 195–206.

Chalmers, D. J. (1995a) Facing up to the problem of consciousness. *Journal of Consciousness Studies*, 2(3), 200–219.

Chalmers, D. J. (1995b) The puzzle of conscious experience. *Scientific American*, December, 62–68.

Chalmers, D. J. (1996) *The Conscious Mind: In Search of a Fundamental Theory*. New York: Oxford University Press.

Crick, F. H. (1994) *The Astonishing Hypothesis: The Scientific Search for the Soul*. New York: Scribner's.

Dennett, D. C. (1991) *Consciousness Explained*. Boston, MA: Little, Brown & Co.

Dreyfus, G., & Thompson, E. (2007) Asian perspectives: Indian theories of mind. In P. D. Zelazo, M. Moscovitch, & E. Thompson (Eds.), *The Cambridge Handbook of Consciousness*. Cambridge: Cambridge University Press, pp. 89–114.

Eddington, A. (1928) *The Nature of the Physical World*. Cambridge: Cambridge University Press.

Freud, S. (2000) *The Unconscious*. London: Penguin Classics. (Original work published 1915).

Giorgi, A. (2009) *The Descriptive Phenomenological Method in Psychology: A Modified Husserlian Approach*. Pittsburgh, PA: Duquesne University Press.

Heisenberg, W. (2000) *Physics and Philosophy: The Revolution in Modern Science*. London: Penguin Classics. (Original work published 1962).

Herbert, N. (1985) *Quantum Reality: Beyond the New Physics*. New York: Doubleday.

Husserl, E. (1970) *The Idea of Phenomenology*. The Hague, The Netherlands: Nijhoff.

Husserl, E. (1980). *Phenomenology and the Foundations of the Sciences*. Boston, MA: Martinus Hijhoff Publishers. (Original work published 1952).

James, W. (1890) *The Principles of Psychology*. New York: Holt.

Krishnamurti, J. (2010) *The Book of Life*. San Francisco: Harper One.

Loy, D. (1988) *Nonduality: A Study in Comparative Philosophy*. New York: Humanity Books.

Lycan, W. G. (1996) *Consciousness and Experience*. Cambridge, MA: MIT Press.

MacKenzie, M. D. (2007) The illumination of consciousness: Approaches to self-awareness in the Indian and Western traditions. *Philosophy East and West*, 57(1), 40–62.

Nagel, T. (1974) What is it like to be a bat? *Philosophical Review*, 4, 435–450.

Parfit, D. (1986) *Reasons and Persons*. Oxford: Oxford University Press.

Penrose, R. (1995) *Shadows of The Mind: A Search for the Missing Science of Consciousness*. London: Vintage.

Puligandla, R. (1970) Phenomenological reduction and yogic meditation. *Philosophy East and West*, 20(1), 19–33.

Rao, K. R. (2011) Cognitive anomalies, consciousness and yoga (vol. XVI, part 1). In D. P. Chattopadhyaya (Ed.), *History of science, philosophy and culture in Indian civilization*. New Delhi, India: New Delhi Centre for Studies in Civilizations/Matrix.

Sartre, J.-P. (1956) *Being and Nothingness: An Essay on Phenomenological Ontology*. New York: Routledge. (Original work published 1943).

Schrödinger, E. (2009) *My View of the World*. Cambridge: Cambridge University Press.

Skinner, B. F. (1953) *Science and Human Behavior*. New York: MacMillan.

Smith, J. A., Flowers, P., & Larkin, M. (2009) *Interpretative Phenomenological Analysis: Theory, Method and Research*. London: SAGE.

Spira, R. (2017) *The Nature of Consciousness: Essays on the Unity of Mind and Matter*. Oakland, CA: New Harbinger Publications.

Tiller, W. A. (1997) *Science and Human Transformation: Subtle Energies, Intentionality and Consciousness*. Walnut Creek, CA: Pavior.

Timalsina, S. (2009) *Consciousness in Indian Philosophy: The Advaita Doctrine of 'Awareness Only'*. Abingdon: Routledge.

Titchener, E. (1901) *An Outline of Psychology*. New York: Macmillan.

van Manen, M. (2017) But is it phenomenology? *Qualitative Health Research*, 27(6), 775–779.

Waite, D. (2007) *Back to the Truth: 5000 Years of Advaita*. Winchester, UK: O Books.

Wallace, B. A. (2000) *The Taboo of Subjectivity: Towards a New Science of Consciousness*. Oxford: Oxford University Press.

Watson, J. (1924) *Behaviorism*. New York: W. W. Norton.

Watts, A. (1976) *Tao: The Watercourse Way*. London: Jonathan Cape.

Watts, A. (2017) *In the Academy – Essays and Lectures*. New York: SUNY Press.

Wundt, W. (1897) *Outlines of Psychology*. Leipzig: W. Engleman.

Zahavi, D. (2005) *Subjectivity and Selfhood: Investigating the First-Person Perspective*. Cambridge, MA: MIT Press.

8

RETHINKING ETHNOGRAPHY WITH PRACTICE THEORY

Engaging with critical theory in qualitative health research

Debbie Hatfield

Introduction

This chapter describes and explains why a focused ethnography was used as a methodological approach for a medical school Doctoral project in the United Kingdom (UK). The study was researching patient and public engagement and involvement (PPEI) for clinical commissioning in the English National Health Service (NHS) and was sponsored by the Higher Education Academy.[1] The focused ethnography provided an opportunity to see the world differently through a practice theory lens. Of interest was the idea of 'meaningful engagement', this being part of the requirements for new Clinical Commissioning Groups (CCGs) which came into being in April 2013; *meaningful engagement with patients, carers and their communities,* (NHS Commissioning Board, 2012). The chapter explores the history of ethnography as well as the strengths and weaknesses of a focused study and why this approach has become increasingly popular in health research. It begins first with some context so that the reader can comprehend the complexity of the landscape which was envisaged as various communities of practice for PPEI. Practice theories and the socio-material are briefly discussed in relation to PPEI for clinical commissioning.

Contextualising the research setting

Public involvement in NHS and (social) care commissioning processes was endorsed with the 'purchaser and provider split' following the NHS and Community Care Act 1990, (Martin, 2009). Organisations purchase services on behalf

---

1   The Higher Education Academy was a national body championing teaching excellence. It is now known as Advance HE – www.advance-he.ac.uk/

of a community from provider organisations such as NHS hospital trusts, the private sector and voluntary and community sector. Purchasing organisations have altered their constitution over the years having been variously called Primary Care Groups, then Primary Care Trusts and now CCGs (Miller et al., 2016). CCGs are statutory NHS bodies led by general practitioners (GPs) which also have a legal duty to support the quality improvement of general practice in primary care (Naylor et al., 2013). They are legally required to involve and engage service users (patients and carers) and the public in the commissioning of services, improving on the design of services and decommissioning services where they are not efficient and effective (Health and Social Care Act, 2012).

In the study, the informants were clinicians (GPs) and service users who were patients and carers, and members of the public (lay representatives) from the local community. Community was defined by the geographical boundaries of the CCG; one urban CCG and another more rural. Given the 25-year history of 'purchasers and providers', the research intended to explore how partnership working with various stakeholders constructed a 'trusted peer' relationship for PPEI for clinical commissioning. This was especially relevant in the post Health and Social Care Act 2012 (HASCA) environment as this legislation had initiated the 200 or so CCGs in England.

Individuals and groups of individuals socially define a reality but so too can organisations. Organisations create a form of reality with specific meanings, shared understandings and values. To identify with those meanings and values and experience that sense of belonging and trust, individuals and groups will align with the organisational discourse. Discourses can be viewed as a form of social practice (Lupton, 2000). They give rise to structures and institutions populated by professional communities that speak a common language and practise according to shared values and policy overseen by legislation (Zeeman, Aranda, & Grant, 2014). The NHS and PPEI for clinical commissioning are an illustration of where such a discourse and policy alignment resides.

The changing nature of engagement and involvement together with the language employed presents challenges for a researcher in this field. Service user and public engagement theory is contested (InHealth Associates, 2014, Tritter, 2009, Checkland et al., 2013, Gibson, Britten, & Lynch, 2012; Phillips, Street, & Haesler, 2016) and the language of citizen participation has 'a remarkable degree of terminological instability' (Stewart, 2013). The lack of consensus together with criticisms of engagement and involvement as unrepresentative (Maguire & Britten, 2017) or tokenistic and encouraging professionally socialised participants (Learmonth, Martin, & Warwick, 2009) prompted a different perspective on PPEI. Instead, to see it as a developing practice or set of practices where meaning and competence change over time together with the materials (physical entities such as surveys, reports and minutes of meetings) used to execute the practices. If the practice changes over time, how has it been carried and how are old and new practitioners (GP commissioners, service users and lay representatives) sustained and recruited? These ponderings shaped the research as practice theory was considered as a lens for illuminating both the methodology and findings.

144 Debbie Hatfield

Practice theories and the socio-material

Practice theories are a sub-type of cultural theory (Reckwitz, 2002). They are concerned with the everyday social practices of life and the tacit knowledge or 'know how' and associated social relations. As a body of ideas, they emerged in the 1970s on the premise that practices consist in organised sets of actions and link together to form wider complexes and constellations (Hui, Schatzki, & Shove, 2017). There is no one unified theory of practice but theories of social practice are popular as part of the contemporary 'practice turn' within the social sciences (Nicolini, 2012, Reckwitz, 2002). Thus, it is a growing field of study with increased interest in the socio-material relations of everyday work and professional learning (Fenwick, 2014; Fenwick & Nerland, 2014a). In addition, within healthcare and organisations and the increasing emphasis on relational approaches to care and leadership, (Cohn, 2015). The appeal of theories of social practice was their application in organisational studies and professional education and practice, including medical education (Goldszmidt & Faden, 2016; Fenwick, 2014).

The writings of Tara Fenwick (Fenwick & Nerland, 2014b; Fenwick, 2014; Fenwick & Nerland, 2014a), Davide Nicolini (2012), Silvia Gherardi (2014; 2016) and Elizabeth Shove (Blue et al., 2014; Shove, Pantzar, & Watson, 2012) influenced the decision to select a practice theory lens for pursuing the research. Re-centring our understandings of social life and associated phenomena as 'practices' places the knowledge and knowing in the doing/activity, as opposed to an acquisition model where knowledge resides in the head of the professional or a person within the organisation (Fenwick & Nerland, 2014a; Gherardi, 2012). Similarly, strategic knowledge which can be thought of as a commodity residing with persons in the work of organisational management is secondary to the knowledge located in the collective, situated activity (Gherardi, 2012). Knowledge acquisition and transfer has been replaced as cognitive attributes of the individual by a participatory mode where practice, knowledge and the environment become entangled in the social and material (Fenwick & Nerland, 2014a). This can dissipate the effects of power and representation in such a way that the ontology or sense of being/reality is altered. The world is viewed in relational terms and knowledge, meaning and discourse are transformed (Nicolini 2012). Shove, Pantzar, and Watson (2012) illustrate this well with their work on understanding change. They argue that unlike other practice theories which focus on reproduction of social life, their slim line version has vast potential for understanding complex change and challenges and could influence public policy. Their interests include public health policy where behaviour change can often focus on individual choice, context, and structural conditions (Blue et al., 2014) depicting the structure and agency dichotomy within the social sciences. How much power or autonomy does the individual have within the structure of healthcare systems for health promotion, for example, giving up smoking or reducing alcohol intake, when set against individual social conditions? A paradigm shift is suggested to focus instead on material and symbolic elements within the 'lives' of social practices (Blue et al., 2014). This leads to exploration of why people are recruited to certain practices and not others and how participation is sustained. Motivation and commitment become the outcomes of engagement rather than the pre-conditions in the above health promotion illustrations (Blue et al., 2014). Practices rather than the practitioners are the units of analysis (Nicolini, 2012). This could equally apply to PPEI practices for clinical commissioning.

Fenwick (2014) similarly explores these ideas where she argues for the growing interest in the socio-material relations of everyday work and why 'matter' matters to medical education. She differentiates between the material and social forces:

Material – the 'everyday stuff of our lives' (Fenwick, 2014) – organic and inorganic such as furniture, pass codes, forms, checklists, minutes, databases, technological. *Social* – symbols and meanings, fears, desires, cultural discourses, politics.

Context is crucial for clinical practitioners when learning in practice and GP clinicians in Lead CCG roles are no different. Metaphors of knowledge acquisition and transfer have been superseded by situated learning where ongoing participation and active engagement within communities need to be understood (Fenwick, 2014).

The research was also informed by practice-based approaches to learning, in particular situated learning theory and Communities of Practice (CoPs) (Wenger, 1998; Wenger-Trayner et al., 2015). The primary focus of Wenger's theory is learning as social participation. As active participants in the practices of social communities we construct our identities in relation to those communities and create a sense of belonging (Wenger, 1998). A CoP does not refer primarily to the group of people participating but the social process of negotiating competence in a domain over time (Farnsworth, Kleanthous, & Wenger-Trayner, 2016). Competence is the dimension of knowing negotiated and defined within a single community of practice by the community members (Wenger-Trayner et al., 2015). It is a learning partnership and has a social dimension to it in that members of the community are perceived as competent or otherwise. 'Domain' is Wenger's preferred term for the area in which a community claims it can legitimately define competence and replaces his original term of 'joint enterprise' (Farnsworth, Kleanthous, & Wenger-Trayner, 2016).

For the purposes of the study the domain was PPEI for clinical commissioning within the landscape of CCGs. The CoPs were the various groups that convene for CCG business that should include and hear the patient and public voice. GP Leads (clinicians), lay representatives and service user representatives are integral to the communities if PPEI practices are to take place. New CoPs are convened according to policy priorities and some may have an intermittent influence depending on NHS commissioning work streams. Examples of communities are the CCG Governing Body, the local authority Health and Wellbeing Board, voluntary and community sector organisations and Patient Participation Groups (PPGs). Although each GP practice[2] should have a PPG not all are actively engaged or involved with clinical commissioning and so some sit outside the domain of practice of PPEI for

2   A GP practice is the physical place where one or more GPs see primary care patients on the GP practice list.

146 Debbie Hatfield

clinical commissioning. Outside of the domain but influencing it and consequently the landscape of CCGs, are other larger and more hierarchical entities. These include the local authority with its remit for population health and (social) care, plus the newer Integrated Care Systems (ICSs) and NHS England which oversees CCGs.

The qualitative researcher curious about the socio-material and situated learning within CoPs for PPEI for clinical commissioning is inevitably drawn to a holistic methodology such as ethnography. Understanding of a phenomenon, as opposed to a population, was being sought. Study participants needed to be in the places where these everyday subjective experiences took place; the CCGs, and where first-hand accounts could be witnessed and heard.

Ethnography – a brief history

Ethnography is central to anthropology and originates from the nineteenth century when the term was used for a descriptive account of a non-Western, 'primitive' culture or community, (Hammersley & Atkinson, 2007). Emanating from the Greek words *ethnos* for 'people' or 'tribe' and *graphia* for 'writing', it simply means 'writing about people' (Scott Jones, 2010). More specifically, *ethnos* refers to people who were non-Greeks. They were strangers, 'other' people and not like the Greeks (Scott Jones, 2010). Ethnographies were compiled by itinerant individuals such as doctors, colonial police officers, travellers and missionaries visiting distant, non-European lands at the end of the nineteenth century. Few would have had any social research training, but they could observe the 'Others' in non-Western, illiterate societies (Scott Jones, 2010; Hammersley & Atkinson, 2007). The ethnographic accounts were then used by 'armchair' anthropologists to compare and contrast the histories and origins of societies and cultures. This was known as 'ethnology' but over time the term lost favour as anthropologists began to conduct their own fieldwork (Hammersley & Atkinson, 2007). Ethnography from the early twentieth century integrated both first-hand accounts and the theoretical and comparative perspectives of culture (Hammersley & Atkinson, 2007). The Polish-born social anthropologist Bronislaw Malinowski was a key figure in this development. His fieldwork in the Trobriand Islands became the template for robust ethnographic practice. It included learning the language of the community under study so as not to rely on interpreters, immersion in the culture by living within, participating in community activities and recording many field notes as well as keeping a field diary to release any emotional tensions (Scott Jones, 2010). He emphasised the importance of a theoretical paradigm and linking social theory to the data.

During the same period, positivism, as a theoretical paradigm, was popular in the social sciences. British and French sociologists favoured the scientific method and empirical study to investigate society in an objective and functionalist manner (Scott Jones, 2010; Hammersley & Atkinson, 2007). Modelled on the natural sciences, this entailed testing theories and hypotheses and generating scientific laws.

Evolutionism and imperialism were also dominant, the former justifying the scrutiny of studying more primitive communities to compare with 'modern' society in the West. Parallels with Charles Darwin's theory of evolution in the animal kingdom encouraged comparison with learning from less complex cultures and adaptation to environment (Scott Jones, 2010). The colonisation of the Asian and African continents was also a persuasive argument for examining 'other' 'barbaric' cultures, thus reinforcing ideas of taking control and ruling over communities or colonies.

The 'Chicago School' rose to prominence after the First World War with its distinctive urban ethnographic fieldwork. Immigration and industrialisation were transforming the North American city. Chicago was like a 'social laboratory' undergoing immense social change, (Scott Jones, 2010). Two founding members of the Department of Sociology at the University of Chicago, Robert E. Park and W. I. Thomas, were influenced by the German phenomenologists Husserl and Schutz and encouraged their students to go out among the people. The 'Others' this time were the immigrants, vagrants and working class in a Western city environment (Scott Jones, 2010). Interpretivism was the methodological lens by which theoretical frameworks were used to explore and explain social action (Scott Jones, 2010). Denzin and Lincoln's generic description of qualitative research helps elaborate:

> Qualitative research is a situated activity that locates the observer in the world. Qualitative research consists of a set of interpretive, material practices that make the world visible. These practices transform the world. They turn the world into a series of representations, including fieldnotes [sic], interviews, conversations, photographs, recordings and memos to the self.
>
> *(Denzin & Lincoln, 2013)*

Interpretivism with its inherent philosophical and sociological ideas, argues that the social world cannot be explained by causal relationships and scientific laws (Hammersley & Atkinson, 2007). Human action is influenced by motives, beliefs, discourse and values which all have social and cultural meanings (Hammersley & Atkinson, 2007). Hence, naturalism encourages the world to be studied in its natural state so that social phenomena as opposed to physical phenomena can be observed. Data are collected with minimal disruption to the social setting. The subjective nature of this reporting has in the past called into question the rigour of ethnographic research (Hammersley & Atkinson, 2007). In the 1960s, issues of representation, power and politics came to the fore (Scott Jones, 2010). How visible were the Others and how empowered were their voices? Ethnographers had not thought about their own influences on their studies and the accounts they wrote or the ethical issues, for example, obtaining consent. Many of the early twentieth century researchers were male and had not considered how subjects might respond to their gender, social class and level of education. This is a point illustrated by the later publication of Malinowski's personal diaries, although these

148 Debbie Hatfield

were not originally intended for public viewing. They revealed misogyny and racism towards the Trobriand Islanders (Scott Jones, 2010). Anthropologists may have been guilty of objectifying their subjects (Cruz & Higginbottom, 2013).

These issues of representation marked a 'turn' in the social sciences with subjectivity, politics and representation becoming much more prominent. This has been described in various ways: the cultural turn, literary turn, post structuralist, post-modern turn (Scott Jones, 2010). Denzin and Lincoln (2013), in describing eight historical moments in North American qualitative research, acknowledge what some described as the crisis of representation (1986–1990) and then refer to a post-modern period (1990–1995) and a methodologically contested present (2000–2010). Qualitative researchers are now confronting a methodological backlash against the evidence-based social movement (Denzin & Lincoln, 2013). Evidence-based medicine (EBM) has been prominent since the early 1990s. It comprises the linear process of asking a clinical question, searching the literature for relevant research articles, critically appraising the articles and then implementing the findings (Greenhalgh, 2018; et al., 1996). Now broadened to include other health and care professionals, managers and lay people it is often described as evidence-based health care (EBHC) (Greenhalgh, 2018). There have been calls to broaden its parameters to include social science methodologies (Greenhalgh, 2018).

The social sciences and humanities are spaces where critical conversations should be taking place; moral discourse on topics such as class, community, nation-states, and globalisation (Denzin & Lincoln, 2013). This post-structural turn also led to an increasing interest in the construction of knowledge and its theory (epistemology) and contextualisation. The contemporary social science researcher must therefore weave and assemble a patched work as in 'bricolage' – quilt making. The researcher becomes a 'bricoleur', borrowing from the many methodological practices of qualitative research (Denzin & Lincoln, 2013).

The rising popularity of ethnographic techniques

There has been increasing interest in ethnographic techniques to research aspects of NHS culture and behaviour. Culture is difficult to define. Silverman (2013) describes it as a common set of beliefs, values and behaviours, whereas Dixon-Woods et al. (2013) liken it to the phrase the 'way we do things round here'. Schein (2004, p. 17) says it is an abstraction; generalised concepts of culture are formulated by taking specific examples and looking for common qualities. He has written extensively about leadership in organisations and defines the culture of a group or organisation as

> a pattern of shared basic assumptions that was learned by a group as it solved its problems of external adaptation and internal integration, that has worked well enough to be considered valid and, therefore to be taught to new members as the correct way to perceive, think, and feel in relation to those problems.
>
> *(Schein, 2004)*

Note within the definition the reference to learning within a group and for new members not unlike CoPs (Wenger, 1998) and newcomers learning by legitimate peripheral participation (Lave & Wenger, 1991).

Ethnographic techniques are not without their critics and a debate in the journal *BMJ Quality and Safety* illustrated the tensions between the 'purists' and the 'pragmatists' (Waring & Jones, 2016). Jowsey (2015) commented on what she perceived as a misrepresentation of ethnography. Observational studies and descriptive statistics do not constitute ethnography. Caution is necessary to avoid separating ethnographic-like methods from the wider methodological principles of ethnography (Waring & Jones, 2016; Jowsey 2016). The methodology requires attention to the underlying concepts including the ontological and epistemological assumptions (Waring & Jones, 2016). However, it may not be possible to include the level of detail required of ethnography in a journal publication and so it could be misconstrued as method by the reader.

There is also increasing pressure in health services research to deliver multi-site findings to a tight time scale and so sustained participant observation typical of ethnography may not be feasible (Waring & Jones, 2016). A recent systematic review on rapid ethnographies refers to the pressures on researchers to generate findings which are actionable and can be used for service improvement (Vindrola-Padros & Vindrola-Padros, 2017). Thus, it creates tension for the researcher between the depth and the breadth of the data and the availability of key informants (Vindrola-Padros & Vindrola-Padros, 2017). The journal editors in the case of the *BMJ Quality and Safety* journal acknowledged the criticisms and emphasised the importance of being clear and consistent with labels in contemporary writing (Dixon-Woods & Shojania, 2016). They also commented on the increasing value of close observation of organisational and clinical practices (Dixon-Woods & Shojania, 2016). Gobo (2008) has remarked that it is as if everything has become 'ethnography' and it is highly fashionable. Given its rising popularity, its broader application in the social sciences to address new contexts and theoretical perspectives since the mid twentieth century, ethnography was a methodology which could help answer the research questions for this study.

Gobo (2008) argues there are at least four components to a methodology in the social sciences:

1. **A pivotal cognitive mode for knowledge acquisition.** This includes observing, listening, questioning, reading, watching and conversing to gather knowledge. One mode maybe more dominant than another but often a knowledge-gathering act is part of a multisensory process. Gobo (2008) uses the example of a doctor palpating a patient's body to 'see' what lies beneath the skin's surface. What the doctor finds on palpation including any tenderness, guarding or rigidity is informed by the patient's response and interaction as part of that practice activity. Similarly, clinical guidelines and policies for performing the procedure. This example illustrates well the 'collective socio-material enactment' (Fenwick, 2014) of the practice where material includes

150 Debbie Hatfield

the body and social the policy imperatives of performing the procedure. Ethnographic methods have been favoured to uncover implicit knowledge and socio-materiality in practice (Kempster, Parry, & Jackson, 2016). 'Observation' is the dominant mode in ethnography but cannot function in isolation without 'listening', 'conversing' and 'questioning'.

2. **A theory of scientific knowledge which comprises a set of assumptions about the nature of reality, the role of the researcher, the tasks of science and the concepts of action and social actor.**

3. Gobo (2008) elaborates on the 'tasks' of science by asking if science should just describe and explain phenomena, intervene to change phenomena or emancipate humankind. Ethnography has typically described and explained. However, Kempster and colleagues (Kempster, Parry, & Jackson, 2016) explore what can be learnt from Strategy-as-Practice researchers to apply to the newer paradigm of Leadership-as-Practice (L-A-P) research. L-A-P was important to this study as it illuminates leadership as a social practice. Citing Orlikowski's summary of three modes of research, Kempster and colleagues (2016) inform how these are useful for the researcher as to the orientation of the research:

    a. The **empirical mode** which examines practice as a phenomenon to find out and understand what practitioners do in practice. It bridges the gap between theory and the lived experience and can generate vast quantities of qualitative data as the researcher engages deeply with the research setting as either a participant or non-participant observer.

    b. The **theoretical mode** where practice is the perspective or lens focusing on the everyday social reality. This mode seeks to develop practice theories that can be used to study organisational activity. It was appropriate to the Doctoral study which sought to theorise patient and public engagement and involvement (PPEI) practices for NHS clinical commissioning. Grounded theory and ethnography are both suitable approaches, but the challenge is what to accept as emergent practice and what to bracket out.

    c. The **meta-theoretical mode** which sees practice as a philosophy and ontologically a social reality. Citing Schatzki (2005) that social life is constituted as 'nexuses of practices and material arrangements', this mode alters the epistemology. Whereas social research draws on a representational epistemology, practice as a philosophy transforms it to a performative epistemology. The knowing comes from directly engaging with the material world.

4. **The range of solutions.** This refers to the 'tricks of the trade' or strategies that you do not find in textbooks but are shared informally amongst fellow researchers as part of the research experience. Sometimes they are made public at conferences and in academic writing. In this study, for example,

access to the research field in one of the case study sites was gained via a commissioning manager who was also a sympathetic postgraduate student.

5. **The procedural steps** which tend to be what many perceive as the 'methodology'; the research design, sampling techniques, research questions, data collection and analysis which are made explicit in the research protocol.

A holistic methodology entails examining context and crystallising data from a range of sources including observations, interviews, documents and discourse. Crystallisation from all the sources helps build new knowledge and theory. The approach acknowledges differences and exceptions in parallel data analysis rather than the congruity of triangulation (Barbour, 2014). Practice is continually emergent and recursive, interacting with the socio-material and so theorising should aim to be plausible and practically adequate (Kempster, Parry, & Jackson, 2016). Ontological position and units of analysis must be clear. Comparative analysis is also useful by case method. Again, drawing on Strategy-as-Practice research Kempster and colleagues (2016) refer to two types of case method named after the researchers. The Eisenhardt (E) case method is of the post positivist paradigm and uses multiple case studies to develop theory that can be tested and generate rules. The second, which was more applicable to this research study, is the Gioia (G) case method. Usually based on a single case for what it can reveal, it is interpretative and not unlike grounded theory. It uses interviews complemented by observations and from the data analysis a process model or theory can be constructed to give an in-depth understanding of the phenomenon. Two CCG case study sites were selected, and the unit of analysis was PPEI practices, that is, where patients and the public were engaged and involved in clinical commissioning with GPs.

Focused ethnography

CCGs are complex organisations different in size and structure, in the way functions are distributed and the roles GPs take (Checkland et al., 2016). There are pressures on the researcher, not least of which is the time it takes to complete the study and the logistics of negotiating multiple geographical sites and obtaining ethical approval from separate commissioning organisations as was the case at the time of the research. Jowsey (2015) refers to a typical time frame of two years but acknowledges ethnography has moved into different spaces, even local, familiar spaces as opposed to the distant Other. The tight time frame of a Doctoral study programme led to consideration of a 'focused ethnography'. It appeared more appropriate for the research questions exploring PPEI in commissioning and leading health and care services in partnership with clinicians, lay representatives and service users.

Muecke (1994) recognised the time constraints for health care professionals who adopt classical ethnography to answer specific questions with a clear purpose and intent. She referred to these accounts as focused ethnographies which are 'programmatic and pragmatic'. They may also be called micro-ethnographies or mini-

152 Debbie Hatfield

ethnographies amongst other terms (Wall 2015). Elsewhere, medical or health ethnographies, have described relationships between cultural beliefs and health behaviours (Higginbottom, Pillay, & Boadu, 2013). There is limited methodological guidance on focused ethnographies but researchers at the University of Alberta in Canada (Higginbottom, Pillay, & Boadu, 2013; Cruz & Higginbottom, 2013; Cruz & Higginbottom, 2015) have published their experiences, compared conventional, anthropological ethnography with focused ethnography and drawn on a number of studies and the expert opinions of Muecke (1994) and Knoblauch (2005). Knoblauch (2005) attributes the term 'focused ethnography' to Otterbien in 1977 with reference to studying a cultural trait. Box 8.1 characterises focused ethnography based on these publications.

More recently, a systematic review of the use of rapid ethnographies in healthcare organisation and delivery included 59 articles using the term focused ethnography (Vindrola-Padros & Vindrola-Padros, 2017). This was defined as 'short-duration fieldwork balanced by data collection and analysis' as part of a typology of rapid ethnographies (Vindrola-Padros & Vindrola-Padros, 2017). Some of the identified potential challenges to inform research questions included breadth versus depth and inability to pick up on changes over time, representativeness and sample size selection leading to only those informants who were available, lone researcher as opposed to multiple researchers with a range of expertise and lack of time for reflexivity of the researcher (Vindrola-Padros & Vindrola-Padros, 2017). The latter is essential if the researcher is to consider how their presence may have influenced the collection and analysis of data.

BOX 8.1 CHARACTERISTICS OF FOCUSED ETHNOGRAPHY

1. Context-specific and focuses on a discrete community, organisation or social phenomena. The phenomena may not be new, but it offers opportunity for 'deep dive' observations across multiple organisational sites (Waring & Jones, 2016).
2. Precise issue or problem, maybe pre-selected with some research questions already formulated. Operates within a closed field as opposed to the open field of conventional ethnography.
3. Time limited, short-term field visits for 'events' as opposed to full immersion in the field.
4. Limited number of participants but they have specific knowledge. They may not all be at one location.
5. Background knowledge outsider perspective (etic view) as opposed to insider knowledge (emic view) of researcher (Higginbottom, Pillay, & Boadu, 2013).
6. Episodic participant observer. Observations may be intermittent or even omitted.

7. Data intensive – a lot of data generated in a short time period. Includes video and audio-recordings and photographs. Recordings as opposed to narrative writings.
8. Data session groups where researchers may gather together to view data collectively, particularly recorded data. Can provide inter-subjectivity and different perspectives as opposed to a single researcher providing a narrative.

Case study design

Having decided a focused ethnography was the preferred methodology, the cases had to be selected. Case study is frequently used to evaluate and research policy implementation (Pope & Mays, 2006). Findings provide an indication of progress and lessons learned and had been used to understand and monitor the development of CCGs (Checkland et al., 2016). PPEI for clinical commissioning and 'meaningful engagement' could be another example of where this could be explored. Despite the Gioia (G) method advocating a single case (Kempster, Parry, & Jackson, 2016), two case study sites were selected because the two CCGs were different in geographical composition.

The case study design was not to test a hypothesis to deduce cause and effect. There was no hypothesis to test as the study was inductive and interpretive. O'Reilly (2009) cites Gary Shank who explains ethnographers use *abductive reasoning*. They make an observation, then gather further evidence from observations, not necessarily in a linear fashion, and then perhaps advance a rule: observation, observation, rule. It is iterative as opposed to the deductive reasoning of rule, observation, result. The CCG settings were for exploring and studying the partnership working for PPEI for commissioning and leading health and care services. This is what Stake (1995) describes as an instrumental case study as opposed to an intrinsic case study. It is a vehicle or means for studying the phenomena in question. Whereas an intrinsic case study is the case itself which is the focus and generalisations and theories are not offered, (O'Reilly, 2009; O'Reilly, 1995).

The cases were a non-probability purposive sample of two CCGs; one urban and one rural. CCGs are unique with respect to their local community profiles but there are national work streams directed by NHS England guidance which all CCGs must implement. NHS England, as an executive non-departmental public body of the Department of Health, oversees the operationalisation of commissioning including the budget and planning. It also has a role in the performance management of CCGs (Petsoulas et al., 2015).

Urban CCGs have similar features and challenges and so too do rural CCGs. The CCGs were selected based on three factors; ethical approval, representativeness of CCG populations and convenience. A suitability profile (Remenyi, 2013)

154   Debbie Hatfield

helped determine the two CCG case study sites in order to bound the research. The CCG case had to be:

Relevant to the research question – engaging service users and the public in commissioning and leading health and care services with clinicians.
Significant in terms of having something important to say – new NHS organisations which reflect the evolving commissioning landscape for health and care services design and delivery.
Geographically accessible location – therefore a non-probability purposive sample.
Amenable to staff co-operation – access to the research field was negotiated via the Patient and Public Engagement Leads for both organisations.

Both cases can be described and bounded but more importantly the *unit of analysis* must be defined and bounded (Remenyi, 2013; Remenyi, 2014). As indicated earlier the unit of analysis was the PPEI practices to elucidate the nature of partnership working and meaningful engagement for commissioning and leading health and care services. Defining the beginning and end of the practices was challenging since various meetings and work streams were ongoing and only snapshots were observed and discussed. There were multiple illustrations given the various meetings and work streams (CoPs) that reported to the CCG Governing Bodies.

Research questions and methods

Focused ethnography, because it is aiming to describe and explain cultural aspects within a group or sub-group, tends to use the first level questions – the 'what?' questions (Higginbottom, Pillay, & Boadu, 2013). Examples might be 'What are the characteristics?' 'What are the shared beliefs?' Secondary questions tend to probe further and explain; 'what helps or constrains?' (Higginbottom, Pillay, & Boadu, 2013). Silverman (2013) refers to an open question for an exploratory study requiring less standardised research instruments. He also links the 'what?' and 'how?' questions to the constructionist model of reality (Silverman, 2013). To operationalise and manage the study, three subsidiary questions in conjunction with the key research question were used and are reproduced below:

What does it mean to work in partnership as clinicians and service users to commission and lead services?

  i. What is the nature of a 'trusted peer' relationship?
 ii. How can relationships be developed to demonstrate effective service user and clinician engagement?
iii. How might this be applied to the topic of patient and public involvement within health care professional education?

The questions centred on exploring the experiences and practices of service users, lay representatives and clinical leaders (GP commissioners) collaborating to commission and lead health and care services. In particular, beliefs and understanding about partnership or working as peers within the changing culture of the NHS in terms of trust relationships. The third subsidiary question was intended to reflect on what the study findings might mean for curriculum development for PPEI in commissioning and leading health and care services.

Three out of the planned four focus groups were completed. Participants were either exclusively service users and lay representatives or exclusively clinicians (GPs) with a leadership role in the CCG. Fifteen non-participant observations were undertaken in the two CCG case study sites together with analysis of documentary sources and material artefacts. The observations were made over the course of 11 months and the meetings observed constituted the regular business of CCGs held every month or two months.

Thirteen interviews were conducted in the two CCG case study sites. The interviewees were Governing Body lay representatives, GP Leads and one service user representative involved with procurement of a service. The interviews were conducted face to face over a period of eight months predominantly on CCG premises. Three interviews were carried out in the homes of participants because it was more convenient for the participant and facilitated discussion that would have been either impossible or time-restricted 'at work'. The duration of the interviews was between 36 and 60 minutes.

Study findings in relation to re-thinking ethnography

Identifying the socio-materialities generated from PPEI practice was important for understanding the meaning of participation within the CCG CoPs and its implications for partnership and learning. This was the purpose of the research questions posed within the focused ethnography. PPEI for clinical commissioning can be re-imagined with practice theory and move beyond the dominant cognitivist and realist accounts. It is not just a product or outcome to be measured for impact. Limited space prevents a full account of the findings here, but re-thinking ethnography with practice theory was highly significant for this Doctoral research study. A conceptual model for learning about and understanding PPEI for clinical commissioning was subsequently formulated from the findings.

Social learning theory and practice theory were used as part of a conceptual and theoretical framework to inform the methodology, data analysis and interpretation. Specifically, CoP theory (Wenger, 1998; -Trayner et al., 2015) was applied to a novel situation; PPEI for clinical commissioning as a domain of practice. The various CCG committees and work streams were re-imagined as functional separate CoPs but also part of a broader landscape of clinical commissioning in the English NHS. They were studied in two CCG case study sites by way of a focused ethnography using four research methods; focus groups, observations, examination of artefacts and interviews. In addition, Wenger-Trayner's idea of 'plug and play'

156 Debbie Hatfield

(Farnsworth, Kleanthous, & Wenger-Trayner, 2016) enabled examination of the data with other practice theories, namely Shove, Pantzar, and Watson (2012) and Raelin's L-A-P movement (2016a and 2016b). Wenger-Trayner acknowledges the evolution of his social learning theory and invites others to apply it to new situations (Wenger-Trayner et al., 2015). This was important given criticisms of CoP theory and its lack of attention to power relations (Fenwick, 2014; Fenwick, 2007).

References

Barbour, R. 2014. *Introducing Qualitative Research: A Student's Guide* (2nd ed.). London: SAGE.

Blue, S., E. Shove, C. Carmona and M.P. Kelly. 2014. "Theories of practice and public health: understanding (un)healthy practices." *Critical Public Health*, 26(1): 36–50.

Checkland, K., P. Allen, A. Coleman, *et al.*2013. "Accountable to whom, for what? An exploration of the early development of clinical commissioning groups in the English NHS." *BMJ Open*, 3(12). doi:10.1136/bmjopen-2013-003769

Checkland, K., I.McDermott, A.Coleman, *et al.*2016. "Complexity in the new NHS: longitudinal case studies of CCGs in England." *BMJ Open*, 6(1). doi:10.1136/bmjopen-2015-010199

Cohn, S. 2015. "'Trust my doctor, trust my pancreas': trust as an emergent quality of social practice." *Philosophy, Ethics, and Humanities in Medicine*, 10(1): 9.

Cruz, E.V. and G. Higginbottom. 2013. "The use of focused ethnography in nursing research." *Nurse Researcher*, 20(4): 36–43.

Denzin, N.K. and Y.S. Lincoln. 2013. *Collecting and interpreting qualitative materials* (4th ed.). Los Angeles: SAGE.

Dixon-Woods, M., R.Baker, K.Charles, *et al.*2013. "Culture and behaviour in the English National Health Servcie: overview of lessons from a multimethod study." *BMJ Quality & Safety*, 23: 106–115.

Dixon-Woods, M. and K.G. Shojania. 2016. "Ethnography as a methodological descriptor: the editors' reply." *BMJ Quality & Safety*, 25: 555–556.

Farnsworth, V., I. Kleanthous, and E. Wenger-Trayner. 2016. "Communities of Practice as a Social Theory of Learning: a Conversation with Etienne Wenger." *British Journal of Education Studies*, 64(2): 139–160.

Fenwick, T. and M. Nerland. 2014a. "Introduction: sociomaterial professional knowing, work arrangements and responsibility: new times, new concepts?" In T. Fenwick and M. Nerland (Eds.), *Reconceptualising professional learning: sociomaterial knowledges, practices and responsibilities*. London: Routledge.

Fenwick, T. and M. Nerland. (eds.) 2014b. *Reconceptualising professional learning: sociomaterial knowledges, practices and responsibilities*. London: Routledge.

Fenwick, T. 2014. "Sociomateriality in medical practice and learning: attuning to what matters." *Medical Education*, 48: 44–52.

Fuller, A. 2007. "Critiquing theories of learning and communities of practice." In J. Hughes, N. Jewson, L. Unwin (Eds.), *Communities of practice critical perspectives*. London: Routledge.

Gherardi, S. 2012. *How to conduct a practice-based study: problems and methods*. Cheltenham: Edward Elgar.

Gherardi, S. 2014. "Professional knowing-in-practice: rethinking materiality and border resources in telemedicine." In T. Fenwick and M. Nerland (Eds.), *Reconceptualising professional learning: sociomaterial knowledges, practices and responsibilities*. Abingdon: Routledge.

Gherardi, S. 2016. "To start practice theorizing anew: the contribution of the concepts of agencement and formativeness." *Organization*, 23(5): 680–698.

Gibson, A., N. Britten, and J. Lynch. 2012. "Theoretical directions for an emancipatory concept of patient and public involvement." *Health (London)*, 16(5): 531–547.

Gobo, G. 2008. *Doing ethnography*. London: SAGE.

Goldszmidt, M. and L. Faden. 2016. "Is medical education ready to embrace the socio-material?" *Medical Education*, 50: 162–164.

Greenhalgh, T. 2018. *How to implement evidence-based healthcare*. Oxford: John Wiley & Sons Ltd.

Hammersley, M. and P. Atkinson. 2007. *Ethnography: Principles in practice* (3rd ed.). London: Routledge.

Health and Social Care Act. 2012. Available at www.legislation.gov.uk/ukpga/2012/7/con tents/enacted [Accessed 18 May 2019]

Higginbottom, G.M.A., J.J. Pillay, and N.G. Boadu. 2013. "Guidance on performing focused ethnographies with an emphasis on healthcare research." *The Qualitative Report*, 18(17): 1–16.

Hui, A., T. Schatzki and E. Shove (eds.). 2017. *The nexus of practices: Connections, constellation, practitioners*. Abingdon: Routledge.

InHealth Associates. 2014. "The engagement cycle." Available at http://engagementcycle. org/ [Accessed 18 May 2019]

Jowsey, T. 2016. "Watering down ethnography." *BMJ Quality & Safety*, 25: 554–555.

Kempster, S., K. Parry and B. Jackson. 2016. "Methodologies to discover and challenge leadership-as-practice." In J.A. Raelin (Ed.), *Leadership-as-practice: theory and application*. Abingdon: Routledge.

Knoblauch, H. 2005. "Focused ethnography." *Forum: Qualitative Social Research*, 6(3): 44.

Lave, J., and E. Wenger. 1991. *Situated learning: Legitimate peripheral participation*. New York: Cambridge University Press.

Learmonth, M., G.P. Martin and P. Warwick. 2009. "Ordinary and effective: The Catch-22 in managing the public voice in health care?" *Health Expectations*, 12: 106–115.

Lupton, D. 2000. "The social construction of medicine and the body." In G.L. Albrecht, R. Fitzpatrick and S.C. Scrimshaw (Eds.), *The handbook of social studies in health and medicine*. London: SAGE.

Maguire, K. and N. Britten. 2017. "How can anybody be representative for those kind of people? Forms of patient representation in health research and why it is always contestable." *Social Science and Medicine*, 183: 62–69.

Martin, G.P. 2009. "Whose health, whose care, whose say? some comments on public involvement in new NHS commissioning arrangements." *Critical Public Health*, 19(1): 123–132.

Miller, R., S. Peckham, A. Coleman, *et al*.2016. "What happens when GPs engage in commissioning? Two decades of experience in the English NHS." *Journal of Health Services Research & Policy*, 21(2): 126–133.

Muecke, M.A. 1994. "On the evaluation of ethnographies." In J.M. Morse (Ed.), *Critical issues in qualitative research methods*. Thousand Oaks, CA: SAGE.

Naylor, C., S. Ross, N. Curry, et al. 2013. *Clinical commissioning groups: supporting improvement in general practice?*London: The King's Fund.

NHS Commissioning Board. 2012. *Clinical Commissioning Group authorisation: a guide for applicants*. NHS England: Author.

Nicolini, D. 2012. *Practice theory, work & organization: an introduction*. Oxford: Oxford University Press.

O'Reilly, K. 2009. *Key concepts in ethnography*. Los Angeles: SAGE.

Petsoulas, C., S. Peckham, J. Smiddy, *et al*.2015. "Primary care-led commissioning and public involvement in the English National Health Service: lessons from the past." *Primary Health Care Research & Development*, 16(3): 289–303.

Phillips, N.M., M. Street and E. Haesler. 2016. "A systematic review of reliable and valid tools for the measurement of patient participation in healthcare." *BMJ Quality & Safety* 25 (2): 110–117.

Pope, C. and N. Mays. 2006. *Qualitative research in health care* (3rd ed.). Oxford: Blackwell.

Raelin, J.A. (ed.) 2016a. *Leadership-as-Practice: theory and application*. Abingdon: Routledge.

Raelin, J.A. 2016b. "Imagine there are no leaders: reframing leadership as collaborative agency." *Leadership*, 12(2): 131–158.

Reckwitz, A. 2002. "Toward a theory of social practices: a development in culturalist theorizing." *European Journal of Social Theory*, 5(2): 243–263.

Remenyi, D. 2013. *Case study research* (2nd ed.; The Quick Guide Series). Reading: Academic Conferences and Publishing International.

Sackett, D.*et al*.1996. "Evidence based medicine: what it is and what it isn't." *British Medical Journal*, 312: 71–72.

Schatzki, T.R. 2005. "The sites of organizations." *Organization Studies*, 26(3): 465–483.

Schein, E.H. 2004. *Organizational culture and leadership* (3rd ed.). New York: John Wiley & Sons.

Scott Jones, J. 2010. "Origins and ancestors: a brief history of ethnography." In J. Scott Jones and S. Watt (Eds.), *Ethnography in social science practice*. London: Routledge.

Shove, E., M. Pantzar, and M. Watson. 2012. *The dynamics of social practice: everyday life and how it changes*. London: SAGE.

Silverman, D. 2013. *Doing qualitative research* (4th ed.). London: SAGE.

Stake, R.E. 1995. *The art of case study research*. Thousand Oaks, CA: SAGE.

Stewart, E. 2013. "What is the point of citizen participation in health care?" *Journal of Health Services Research & Policy*, 18(2): 124–126.

Tritter, J.Q. 2009. "Revolution or evolution: the challenges of conceptualizing patient and public involvement in a consumerist world." *Health Expectations*, 12(3): 275–287.

Vindrola-Padros, C. and B. Vindrola-Padros. 2017. "Quick and dirty? A systematic review of the use of rapid ethnographies in healthcare organisation and delivery." *BMJ Quality & Safety*, 27: 321–330.

Wall, S. 2015. "Focused ethnography: a methodological adaptation for social research in emerging contexts." *Forum: Qualitative Social Research*, 16(1): Art1.

Waring, J. and L. Jones. 2016. "Maintaining the link between methodology and method in ethnographic health research." *BMJ Quality & Safety*, 25(7): 556–557.

Wenger, E. 1998. *Communities of practice: learning, meaning, and identity*. Cambridge: Cambridge University Press.

Wenger-Trayner, E., M. Fenton-O'Creevy, S. Hutchinson, *et al*. (eds.). 2015. *Learning in landscapes of practice: boundaries, identity and knowledgeability in practice-based learning*. Abingdon: Routledge.

Yin, R.K. 2014. *Case study research: design and methods* (5th ed.). Los Angeles: SAGE.

Zeeman, L., K. Aranda and A. Grant. 2014. "Queer challenged to evidence-based practice." *Nursing Inquiry*, 21(2): 101–111.

9

AUTOETHNOGRAPHY

Alec Grant

Introduction

This chapter is meta-autoethnographic to the extent that it speaks to auto-ethnography and autoethnographic work in an autoethnographic way. I'm proud of the contribution my colleagues and I have made in recent years to raising the profile of the autoethnography in the UK (Short et al., 2013) and internationally (Turner et al., 2018). In what follows, I draw largely but not exclusively on my own single- and co-authored writing and will provide some illustrative quotes, mostly from this healthcare-related work, in italicised text boxes. In sometimes addressing you, the reader, in the second person, I want to pull you into my narrative so that you can consider its relevance for your own life and healthcare research.

I'll begin by defining autoethnography, setting out its key characteristics, forms, and demands on the researcher. Next, I'll look at the relationship between the autoethnographic self and culture, and the political implications of this relationship. This will pave the way for an exploration of some key governing philosophical principles shaping the approach. After describing its benefits, I'll discuss issues around evaluation and dissemination. My response to some the main criticisms levelled at autoethnography will bring the chapter to its conclusion.[1]

---

1   Since autoethnography is an evolving, and theoretically and methodologically rich transdisciplinary methodology within qualitative inquiry, my focus in this chapter is necessarily selective. I make no attempt to descriptively exhaust all of its variants, and theoretical and empirical possibilities, but invite you explore these areas yourself by reading the work I have cited. Nor do I cover the complexities of ethical challenges posed by autoethnographic inquiry in this chapter. These are always implicitly present in autoethnographic writing, as you will realise from reading the quotes from my own work, below. I will explore some of them in the Chapter Eleven, in the context of reflexivity.

160 Alec Grant

Defining and unpacking autoethnography

Autoethnography is

> research, writing, and method that connect the autobiographical and personal
> to the cultural and social. The form usually features concrete action, emotion,
> embodiment, self-consciousness, and introspection...[and] claims the conven-
> tions of literary writing.
>
> *(Ellis 2004 in Grant et al., 2013, p. 2)*

In unpacking Ellis's definition, I think it's important to stress to you that the critical
relationship between autobiography and the sociocultural world is key to understanding the approach. Charles Wright Mills (1959) argued for the development of
the 'sociological imagination', to turn the private issues of social researchers into
public concerns. This requires us to be philosophically, politically, theoretically and
empirically savvy about the relationship between our biographies and the socio-
cultural historical periods in which these are situated. Autoethnographic inquiry
calls out for such a level of critical awareness, to contest the history that usually
goes on behind our backs (Denzin, 2018). Autobiographical writing of self and
others, cultural interrogation, and analysis all need to be present in work purport-
ing to be autoethnographic. I will stress again near the end of the chapter that the
approach is expressly *not* simply one of telling stories.

Autoethnographic forms

You also need to know that autoethnography can take many forms. Among my
past doctoral students and others I have taught and/or mentored are, for example,
those working in film (Young, 2013, 2015), autoethnodrama (Moriarty, 2015), and
fine art (Diab, 2017). All come to realise fairly quickly that it's important to work
hard at the craft. I always urge those who want to become narrative (article and
book/chapter) autoethnographers to read and write a lot. If you want to do autoethnographic performance in other ways, go to see lots of films, plays, or art work.
However, don't imagine that art-based and narrative autoethnographies are
mutually exclusive areas. Norman Denzin (2018) reminds us that all autoethnographic work is *performance*; so, for example, filmic, dramatic and fine art modality
autoethnographies can be combined with narrative, and vice versa (see e.g. Moriarty, 2015; Diab, 2017).

Autoethnography and narrative writing

If your intention is to become a narrative autoethnographer – someone who writes
autoethnography – it's unwise to assume that you already have the ability to
express yourself in the engaging and evocative way that the methodology demands.
Look again at Ellis's definition above: '... [and] claims the conventions of literary

writing.' Autoethnographic writing should not be assumed to be a vehicle to present knowledge after the fact, as in more traditional forms of qualitative inquiry. Writing *is* the vehicle with which you will create knowledge, so you'll need to have a performance set of *writing*, not *writing up*. This requires you to always start writing early, avoiding the constant deferral of fingers on keyboard. And it's important to practice, practice, practice! I urge you to enrol on creative writing and poetry classes to become more sensitive to, and skilled in, the creative and nuanced uses of language.

As a narrative autoethnographer, I practice what I preach. I have taken creative writing classes, and my work experiments with narrative and poetic form (see Box 9.1).

BOX 9.1 MY BROTHER WAS VERY FAT

My brother was very fat.
He had a fat wife.
They fed on fat ideas, which they spewed up again and again.
They swallowed everything.

Fat words popped out of their fat mouths,
Faster than fat food.
Clogging up the space between us
forever.

Undigested half-truths,
plump lies,
celebratory cakes.

Gorging on their unacknowledged mediocrity,
their recipe for knowing me
was always minus my ingredients.

(Sorly et al., in press)

I read a prodigious number of books. This includes auto/biographical work, literary fiction in the form of short stories and novels, poetry, philosophy texts, and work pertaining to narrative, human and social science theory, and the human condition. I'm also always writing. This involves me in drafting, re-drafting, cutting, revising and experimenting, until I get to the point where I don't think I can improve on a text.

162 Alec Grant

My single- and joint-authored work is always critically culturally-interrogative. It includes short stories (e.g. Grant, 2017, 2018b; Grant & Zeeman, 2012), meta-stories – stories about stories employing narrative and poetic form (Sorly, et al., in press), and autotoethnographies about teaching, mentoring and co-publishing in mental/health-care and beyond (Grant, 2017; Grant, in press; Klevan et al., in press).

Culture

You may be asking at this point, what then is the relationship between the autoethnographic self and 'culture'? With my colleagues, I follow others in arguing that culture can be regarded in a broad and comprehensive way – as socially and materially shared, linguistic, representational and activity-based life practices (Grant, 2018a; Grant et al., 2013, 2015). To put it another way, 'culture' refers to the usually taken for granted ways we live our lives, and maintain our beliefs, assumptions and life and community allegiances. From this perspective, culture flows through self, and vice versa.

An important critical function of autoethnography is therefore to reflexively expose cultural 'elephants in rooms'. I'm using this metaphor to refer to those normative everyday practices and assumptions that lend themselves to, and sometimes cry out for, robust scrutiny and critique, but which are often insufficiently explored and simply regarded as natural and reasonable parts of life. In resisting this normative tendency, the autoethnographer fulfils the important role of cultural trickster or cultural conscience agent (see Box 9.2).

BOX 9.2 OTHERING

I . . . experience . . . the contradictions between professional and educational rhetoric and displays of disparaging and 'othering' accounts of students and qualified staff about the people they purport to be in the business of caring as deeply offensive. They could be talking about me in my days as an acute ward patient. . . . However, I am by no means free of blame in this regard. At a recent social event, I spent the evening with a group of mental health nurse educators. Over dinner, we shared nostalgic stories of our times as student mental health nurses back in the 1970s. One of my companions described the first time he met a patient after the latter's recent lobotomy. His graphic description of how this changed the shape of the patient's head and facial features is met with guffaws by my companions. I joined in with the laughter.

Later at my home, I become pre-occupied with lots of conflicting thoughts, and feel a mixture of mild self-disgust and bitter irony over . . . my collusion in storying patients in 'othering' and abusive ways. . . . I had also shared one or two patient anecdotes, breaking my own rules in the interests of maintaining bonhomie, and co-constructing a group identity through the use of humour.

(Grant, 2016c, p. 197)

As the above quote illustrates, it's important to stress to you that we are all inscribed within culture(s), rather than culture being 'out there', separate from us. Culture is performed and material; we *do* culture in our thinking, dreaming, loving, hating, working, sleeping, dressing, and in all other aspects of our lives. Autoethnographers (who are as it were are never off duty) follow the qualitative inquiry maxim of finding the strange in the culturally familiar. However, they do this in arguably more astute, critical, and personally and relationally significant ways than is the case in among qualitative researchers more generally. Cultural practices are never innocent, and some taken-for-granted cultural assumptions practices are downright weird aren't they (think about your own professional and wider life cultures for a moment)?

Despite the strangeness of some of our assumptions, as narrators of our lives we all generally tend to pull on dominant and taken-for-granted cultural stories to co-create our own. I will talk in greater theoretical depth about this issue later, but for the moment I simply ask you to think about the dangers of regarding those dominant narratives as 'just so', 'right and proper' and *the truth*.

The personal is political

The interrogation of the ways in which taken-for-granted master narratives represent life has political importance for those of us who feel we (and this may include you?), or the people we research with, have been culturally excluded and marginalised. Such dominant narratives of how life *is* or is *supposed to be* are often at odds with our lived-experiences. Autoethnography therefore also challenges those dominant cultural stories and practices normally assumed to be benign – by no means a pain-free endeavour (see Box 9.3).

BOX 9.3 WHOSE STORY IS IT?

In my late middle age, I contacted the school secretary from the small rural Scottish town where I spent the first 16 years of my life. From this phone call I was routed to one of the teachers who obligingly sent me some spare copies of my old school magazine. Published annually, they covered the years between 1948 . . . and 1968, . . . the year I left the town. They were to make poignant reading, but it took me a while to open them up and look inside. I felt a surge of familiar anxiety as I unwrapped the parcel and once again saw "Age pro viribus", the school motto, emblazoned on the yellow cover of each magazine. Inside the pages were illustrated stories. Stories of the past. Stories of my time, from my time, kind of.

Age pro viribus: In all that you do, do your best. . . . I felt self-conscious as I looked at the pile of time-worn magazines. Under scrutiny perhaps? There was a meta-voyeuristic feel to the idea of wanting to look inside the pages, knowing that some people from the town knew about my interest and request (made for "scholarly purposes") and were perhaps curious about this. News travels fast in a small town, population 1,400.

When I eventually looked inside the magazines, I saw faces and names of people I remembered. All smiling, all pristine, from more than four decades back. . . . As I read and re-read the magazines, I was reminded of a belief I had as a youngster: that there was only room for success stories in their pages. Depending on how they are read, photos of, and stories by and about, well-turned out adolescents signify a particular kind of cultural narrative. Complexity and difference are effaced, airbrushed out. Photos of pupils in their school uniforms are testimony to homogenization, to single stories, to monocultures. Age pro viribus. Cultural conformity (or at least the appearance of it) promises rewards. No dissenters graced the pages.

And the future focus was in keeping with this style of representation. The former pupil lists spoke of success and conformity; of tidied up, sanitized representations of human lives. All was achievement piled on achievement. Promotion, degrees, higher degrees, more sporting successes. All were happy lives, marriages, and babies. Even death was purified. People had "nice ends" and "passed peacefully away". No nastiness here. No alcoholics, broken marriages, broken people, broken lives.

And there were bigger stories. The school magazine down the years told tales of inter-generational dynasties. Dynasties which smelled like roses and did not wilt (or die nastily). The promise of eternal respectable certainty shone out from pages produced annually and circulated internationally for the benefit of ex-pat readers.

And the pages communicated an assumption about the school, as an organization, which complemented the above. In magazine after magazine its image was presented as benign. A warm and cheerful place. A harmless bricks and mortar backdrop to gainful, happy and productive activity in learning and on the track and field. Age pro viribus.

But there were losers, and the local graveyard in my town tells part of this story (although of course no headstone is testament to this). My mother was buried there in 1974 after she hanged herself.

(Grant & Zeeman, 2012, pp. 3–4)

Autoethnography and the methodological politics of the academy

'The personal is always political' is a truism not a posture slogan. It applies to you and your situated research practices. With regard to the politics of scholarship, I have argued with others that autoethnography represents sustained resistance against the kinds of mainstream healthcare research work expected by corporate, new public managed, neoliberal universities, where positivist assumptions and practices dominate (Grant 2018a; Klevan et al., in press). Against this oppressively conformist backdrop, there has been a recent call (which I will speak more about later) for qualitative inquiry more generally to breach strict methodological boundaries in moving more towards experimentalism and new onto-epistemological practices (Grant, 2018a). This is essential in challenging the anti-intellectual and creativity-constraining environments that many of us palpably experience in the healthcare departments of our 'New Public Managed' or 'Neoliberal' universities (Grant, 2018a; Klevan et al., in press; Klevan et al., in review), and in related healthcare publishing, journal article reviewing and editorial practices (Grant 2016a).

In embracing autoethnography as a radical alternative to realist-positivist social and human science inquiry, many researchers have thus understandably come to reject the research and publishing assumptions and practices associated with more traditional qualitative approaches. This includes privileging the researcher over the subject, an over-concern with method at the expense of story, pre-occupations with outmoded conceptions of validity, truth and generalisability, and a relative lack of attention paid to social injustice in the form of cultural power (Grant 2016b, 2018a; Grant et al., 2013, Klevan et al., in press, in review). In my case, this rejection has helped me to engage more with New Materialist thinking which, because it embraces posthumanist philosophy, accords agency to non-human animals and material objects (Grant 2016b, 2017, 2018b). I will illustrate this point from my work in my next chapter in this volume, *The Reflexive Autoethnographer*.

Philosophical background

This picture of rejection relates to critical tensions emerging in the philosophy of science governing qualitative research in the second half of the twentieth century. Included among these are the emergence of the Postmodern, Poststructural and, more recently, New Materialist paradigms.[2] These pose a challenge to many of the reality and knowledge claims, and representational and dissemination practices, of traditional qualitative approaches (Grant, 2018a; Turner et al., 2018).

These critiques are in turn associated with the shifting landscape of qualitative inquiry since the 1980s. Norman Denzin and Yvonna Lincoln (2000) describe 'seven moments' characterising the contours of the development of twentieth- and twenty-first century qualitative inquiry. I want to stress to you at this point the importance of thinking of Denzin and Lincoln's key moments as conceptual heuristics. They should be regarded as enduring tendencies in qualitative inquiry rather than linearly-emerging, historical periods in its development.

The first two moments capture the power of traditional objectivist-realist, or positivist, assumptions informing qualitative approaches. The five subsequent

2   It is beyond the scope of this chapter to explain and discuss these paradigms. You can see it in poststructuralist and postmodernist autoethnographic action in Grant (2013) and in some of the chapters in Turner et al. (2018). For a more in-depth exploration of the role and function of paradigms in qualitative inquiry, see successive editions of Denzin and Lincoln's edited SAGE text, *Handbook of Qualitative Inquiry*.

166 Alec Grant

moments have direct relevance for the development and significance of auto-ethnography. The *third moment* of 'blurred genres' refers to the dissolving of the boundaries between the social sciences and the humanities. Sparkes (2002) argues that science and art, thus fact and fiction have softened to the extent that writing and other representational approaches which would have previously been regarded as inferior by both social research and arts communities is now made possible. This is played out in the *fifth, sixth* and *seventh moments*, in, respectively, experimental, postexperimental and future forms of representational practices, including fictional, poetic and multimedia ethnographic work.

The *fourth moment*, focuses attention on researcher writing practices. Marcus and Fischer (1986) described a 'crisis of representation' arising from a growing uncertainty about how to describe social reality adequately. A lack of faith set in about the implicit promise of qualitative social research to accurately, objectively and appropriately mirror a passive social world, waiting for its expert gaze.

The crisis of representation brought with it postmodernism's defining scepticism towards 'grand' narratives, or 'master stories', in favour of autoethnographic local stories which often challenge the truth claims of master stories. Master stories are taken-for-granted, all-encompassing narratives about the world or aspects of it, which often disadvantage people as much as they provide them with positive social identities. Local stories, written by autoethnographers about specific events, testify to such disadvantage.

In healthcare, for example, the master story of 'mental illness' saturates the public, professional and academic consciousness. It is accepted as a cultural fact by many, signifying a binaried distinction between those who 'suffer from' 'mental illness' and those who don't. Although this master story satisfies many, it equally often results in biographical violence for others in the form of 'narrative entrapment'. In a (local story) relational autoethnography, my co-writers and I used this term to bring attention to our toxic cultural experience of being caught up in stigmatising stories while patients in acute psychiatric wards (see Box 9.4).

BOX 9.4 NARRATIVE ENTRAPMENT

By the time I was admitted to hospital in London, I felt in some ways that I had used up all of my narratives, but still I tried to talk about my existential and emotional difficulties with the staff on the acute ward. Most of the time, their non-verbal expressions indicated levels of boredom that increased in direct proportion to my attempts at repeated clarification and re-clarification of what was going on for me. As a result of this, my feelings of personal worthlessness and vulnerability worsened. I felt, and was, chastised, shamed and humiliated. The worst example of this was when a young, male staff nurse came into my room late one morning. I had no idea what time it was and had just woken up, multiple hypnotics and trancs contributing to me oversleeping. Clearly irritated, he shouted at me: 'Don't you want to get better? Get up, you cxxt'. . . . I felt increasingly caught up in the stories told about me by staff, particularly what was written about me in the nursing and medical notes. One entry described me as having a personality disorder. This jarred with my wish not to be, after Stockwell, the 'unpopular patient'. I wanted to be regarded in a fair way and be validated as a person, as opposed to being in receipt of, in Goffman's sense, a spoilt identity that took no account of contextual factors.

(Grant et al., 2015, pp. 282–283)

Scepticism towards grand or master narratives does not imply disbelief or dismissal of them. It means critical interrogation of their claims, assumptions and onto-epistemological bases (what is pre-supposed about reality, knowledge and knowing). I hope you develop such scepticism, because many mainstream qualitative researchers appear deficient in it. For example, I have met, read and peer reviewed the work of some phenomenological researchers who seem to wholeheartedly and un-critically believe in the 'researcher as mirror of the world' metaphor. So, not surprisingly, quite a number of their articles are atheoretical, apolitical and lacking in context, attracting the criticism that this work displays naïve realism through simply and unreflexively promoting whatever cultural status quo marks the period it was written in.

In a more disturbing way, such assumed researcher authority and neutrality – held across many methodological approaches, not just phenomenology – promotes a form of implicit othering, with researchers often seeming in their writing to transcend and grossly simplify the world and their participants. In conventional qualitative inquiry, examples of representations of people stripped of their socio-cultural contexts are commonplace. Strings of quotes are used to support researcher themes which, too frequently and in the absence of adequate methodological explanation or justification, appear to magically 'emerge from the data'. As a critical autoethnographer this fascinates me and compels me to write (see Box 9.5).

BOX 9.5 CONVENTIONAL QUALITATIVE INQUIRY

[I]t seems to me that taken for granted binaries prevail in mental health nursing phenomenological-humanist qualitative inquiry. The frequent use of terms such as 'self' and 'identity' usually implies coherent identities separate from the world which is assumed to be outside of, and relatively unrelated to, self. The implicitly 'mentally well' are divided from the 'mentally ill', as are the (well) researchers from (ill) participants. The absence of a critically reflexive commentary around the assumptions underpinning these terms in the context in which they appear makes it seem as if their use is unproblematic. In this regard, readers of these articles are implicitly invited to take for granted that these assumptions and terms are necessary and sufficient to accurately and fairly

168 Alec Grant

> represent the world, topic, and people under discussion, in ways that transcend culture, time, and place.
>
> Related to the use of these terms in research narratives and to the kinds of worlds they speak into existence, people represented in these articles are often portrayed as existing in special kinds of macroisolation units devoid of real-life contexts. At an environmental level, participants and researchers are portrayed as separated and insulated from messy and contradictory human organizational and social cultures. Both groups apparently often live in power-neutral or power-silent, apolitical environments, where healthcare organizations are represented as benign unproblematic backdrops to practice.
>
> *(Grant 2016b, p. 291)*

The narrative turn and narrative healing

The above suggests a need to shift from a narrow range, inflexible conception of what should constitute scholarly work to a representational pluralism which honours the rich, politicized and emancipatory, contexts of people's lives. The pluralist agenda of what is often described as the 'narrative turn' in social inquiry recognises and promotes multiple forms of such storied experience. Exemplified in autoethnography, the narrative turn signals the increasing celebration of reflexive, subjective, first person, culturally engaged stories which aim more for *connection* with readers than *pedagogic instruction*. Through such connection, collective and individual healing can be both achieved and represented(see Box 9.6).

BOX 9.6 NARRATIVE RECOVERY

A significant strand on my road to recovery was being allocated a CPN who worked within a recovery value system and who seemed to want to patiently listen to me and help me to explore my own recovery path. Through dialogue with this CPN, whom I eventually came to trust, I found therapeutic value in beginning to understand what my experiences meant and what was happening to me. This contrasted with years of being simply given a diagnosis and told I should accept treatment provided on the basis of mental health professionals knowing what was best for me and having any questioning by me of either diagnosis or treatment . . . regarded as further signs of illness.

All of this contributed to me feeling helped as opposed to simply managed, and as a result I gradually came to terms with the loss of my career and embraced the need to change direction. I began service user project work and have come to regard this as central to my recovery. Hearing the stories of others has made me realize the resilience and courage needed for recovery in the face of a largely unsympathetic and stigmatizing society. This has helped

me in the transition from feeling ashamed about having a mental health problem to feeling proud to be a member of the mental health recovery community . . .

I have been able to reclaim my academic skills in contribution to the
improvement of mental health service provision while working with mental
health nursing and clinical psychology students. Telling and retelling my story,
verbally and in print, has enabled me to gain an increasingly richer understanding of my own experiences and confidence in them. No longer afraid of
people's reactions to my stories, including mistrusting them, this consolidates
for me the notion of shared/community story telling as central in narrative
recovery, in terms of being therapeutic and exploratory in making sense of the
past and creating a narrative template for now and the future. My story is
changing and developing, as I am. I have also found it hugely therapeutic to
have the opportunity to challenge the 'official' story about me that has been
told and continues to be told in my medical record, but which I have no part in
telling.

(Grant et al., 2015, p. 282)

Lives that have suffered narrative interruption – assaults to tacitly held, coherent
stories about their forward movement – can progress on the basis of new stories
which function as a kind of moral compass for how they should be lived. Such
writing can help individuals make better sense of their pasts and re-focus on their
futures, and can also mobilise readers who connect with such stories to join, in
solidarity, emerging communities of meaning making (Frank, 2010; Grant &
Leigh-Phippard, 2014; Grant & Zeeman, 2012; Grant et al., 2012, 2015).

This suggests that there's a kind of moral order to stories, which has implications
for their power and significance as healing tools. We narrate our lives in retrospect,
in order to give our lives coherence. Arguably, the more coherent our stories, the
better our emotional and (in a broad sense) spiritual health. The fact that we can
pull on 'off the peg' stories can make us lazy, thoughtless and morally compromised. In our lives and writing we can, as Minnich (2017) argues, draw on stock
clichés in a thoughtless way – at worst in the service of rule following. You might
find it instructive to keep your eye out for healthcare qualitative work that per-
petuates oppressive service level practices, through simply uncritically regurgitating
the vocabulary of those practices.

Benefits of autoethnography: why do it?

By this stage in the chapter, you may have asked yourself the above question. Or
you may have already begun to answer it? In line with everything I've written thus
far, Stacy Holman Jones and her colleagues (2013) argue that autoethnographic
work is beneficial for four reasons. The first is in *disrupting norms of research practice*

170 Alec Grant

and representation. From a conventional qualitative inquiry perspective, if a person had breast cancer and was doing research on that topic, writing about their experiences may be seen to be biasing the topic.

The second is in *working from insider knowledge.* Autoethnographers value what are often called 'thick', or highly detailed, descriptions of cultural experiences, important in bringing topics alive. Unfortunately, as argued above, the complexity and fragility of life is often inadequately captured or even silenced by dominant cultural master stories.

The third benefit is the significance of autoethnography in *manoeuvring through pain, confusion, anger and uncertainty in order to make life better.* Many auto-ethnographers write about their experiences when their worlds fall apart and master stories don't account for, or contradict, those experiences. Such writing will com-plement other similar stories, which directly relates to the fourth benefit. This is breaking silence through the reclamation of voice, or 'writing to right' through community storying against dominant cultural stories.

Finally, Holman Jones and her colleagues argue that autoethnography is bene-ficial in *making work accessible.*[3] Academic writing generally is often criticised for being jargon laden, elitist and impenetrable, appealing mostly to other academics. One of the purposes of autoethnography is therefore to create work that speaks to people in general. The inclusion of life stories that, hopefully, a range of audiences can relate to is thus important in autoethnographic work (see Box 9.7).

BOX 9.7 DRINKING TO RELAX

His shoes crunch the shingle on the short path as he slowly lumbers towards his council house. At sixty, looking seventy-five, he carries the sadness of four decades of bad marriage and chronic unfulfillment. Stooped, obese, arterio-sclerotic, hungover, labored breathing in time with short pinch-toe gait, he trudges reluctantly to the front door. Anticipatory defensive anger builds and quickly turns his face from default red to puce. Three short steps to go as, sweating, he prepares for the onslaught. Key in the lock now. Turn slowly. Open door quietly. There she is. Dash meets Peg. Peg meets Dash. As usual. Only this time Peg is not ranting vitriol at full volume. Only this time Peg is dead dead not dead drunk. Purple face meets purple face. Two yards from the front door, feet off the ground, her body swings obscenely in this final Fuck You goodbye moment.

(Grant, 2018b, pp. 33–34)

---

3   The representational practices of autoethnographers are challenging in this area. They have to write in ways that reveal the stuff of ordinary life, while being careful about uncritical displays of naïve realism. So they have a double task: to reflexively write about ordinary life which critically addressing its cultural contingency. Hearts needs to be accompanied by heads.

However, I think there's a fifth benefit which undermines the assumption of universal cultural recognition. This is in work that is at first culturally unfamiliar but comes to prove mutually beneficial through developing a connection between audiences and its producers. I sometimes engage with autoethnography that takes me a long while to 'get'. It may have been crafted by people who are much younger than me, of a different gender, sexuality, ethnicity, or geographical location, who have cultural insider awareness that I lack. I may also experience such work as off putting. Sometimes this is because of its topic and/or the modalities and tropes through which it is expressed. When I get to the point where I get something out of it, I'm reminded of how autoethnography can help people develop their levels of *cultural appreciation*. Climbing out of our cultural boxes requires perseverance, and leaps in empathy and imagination.

Challenges for autoethnographers: evaluation and dissemination

Evaluating autoethnography

BOX 9.8 FUNCTION OR FLAVOR?

The flat piece, a cold dinner, is forced down, taken in with little pleasure. It lacks the heat of the chef's passions, the chef's sensuous self who knows, without spice, all is bland. The engaging piece makes each mouthful worthy of comment, encourages lingering, savouring, remembering. In its presence, I want to invite my colleagues and students to enjoy its flavors.

(Pelias, 2011, p. 666)

As you engage with them, you might find yourself wondering how to judge the quality of autoethnographies. Andrew Sparkes (2018, in press) argues that attempts to evaluate qualitative work generally often use criteria lists. With specific reference to autoethnography, Holman Jones et al. (2013) for example propose: purposefully commenting on/critiquing cultural practices; making contributions to existing research; Embracing vulnerability with a purpose; and creating a reciprocal relationship with audiences in order to compel a response.

How the criteria characteristics of any evaluation list is played out in practice is up for grabs, however. Any list should be provisional, flexible and open-ended, because the criteria used to judge an autoethnographic piece are always contingent, changing according to context and purposes – both of the piece itself and those judging it. An autoethnographic text judged favourably at one point in time and place may be judged harshly at another. Moreover, the production of novel,

172   Alec Grant

innovative autoethnographic work may not fit well with existing list criteria. Lists are forever out of date.

Sparkes (in press) points out that a major potential and actual problem with evaluative lists, therefore, is that failing to recognise their cultural contingent nature might result in them being used in a rigid, prescriptive and normative manner to police the boundaries of autoethnographic practice. In the noble attempt to ensure rigour, rigour mortis might ensue.

Disseminating autoethnography

Such boundary policing also detracts from, and fails to take into account, variable reader judgements in the dissemination of autoethnographic work.

BOX 9.9 MORAL EVALUATION

[A]utoethnographic stories, like all stories, are inevitably experienced by their audiences on a spectrum. Some audiences may find some stories meaningful and helpful, in contrast to others read as toxic and offensive. Tales that evoke various shades of indifference and positive and negative resonance reside somewhere in the middle of this spectrum. Judgements about whether auto-ethnographic stories are 'good' or 'bad' are usually made on the basis of indi-vidual cultural taste, narrative sophistication and audience consensus... Autoethnography is not just about writing texts which are assumed by their authors to have universal resonance, appeal and utility.

(Grant, 2018, pp. 109–110)

The meaning gaps between autoethnographers and their audiences interests me. Clearly, people may experience the stories they read in ways that jar with their implicitly held world views. Have you ever had that experience? Roland Barthes (1977) asserted that it is language which speaks, not the author. Bronwyn Davies and Rom Harre (1990) argued similarly – that words speak us in terms of our positioning within, and availability of discourses. Words are all we have, and words are up for grabs. Words can unite us. Equally, words can drive meaning wedges between us, forcing us apart.

Standard criticisms of autoethnography and rejoinders to these

This observation applies to the collective words that constitute the autoethno-graphic genre in its totality. In bringing this chapter to a close, you may be inter-ested in reading about the twitter trolling experienced by my autoethnographic colleague, Elaine Campbell (2017). The unpleasant accusations expressed in the tweets sent to her exemplify some of the standard criticisms levelled at auto-ethnographers and their work.

Campbell was told that her work amounted to 'diddling your pet hamster'. The sexual symbolism employed here implies that autoethnographers are nothing more than textual masturbators; self-indulgent narcissists engaged in trivial 'me-search'. Rebutting this charge, Laurel Richardson (1997, 2001), has written extensively about the political significance of the attempt to suppress subjective voices in the academic literature. Given that it's impossible to create authentically objective research, with no trace of the author/s, researchers who write from an explicitly emotional 1st person stance call on readers to feel, react, discover and care. Far from the subjective constituting a contaminant in qualitative inquiry, it can powerfully bring it to life by, as Moriarty (2014) puts it, 'leaving the blood in'.

Campbell's work was further trivialised as just 'stuff that happened to me', the implicit accusation here being that autoethnography is unscientific. Sara Delamont (2009), among others argues that personal narrative is not a proper concern of social science, and researchers should therefore keep themselves separate from their research. These criticisms are inappropriate on two counts, which I argued earlier. Autoethnography is expressly *not* just about telling personal stories. It is always mediated by a commitment to contextualised cultural interrogation. Moreover, in terms of its representational practices, autoethnography is a blurred genre approach, marrying the social and human sciences with the humanities through the use of drama, fiction, and broader devices and tropes from across the arts disciplines. Contrary to Delamont's (2009) related accusation that autoethnography lacks intellectual rigour, if you engage with it seriously you will find that the task of crafting autoethnography demands high and sustained levels of deep scholarly introspection and reflexivity.[4]

Finally, Campbell was asked 'I get it's writing about yourself, but what if you don't have anything interesting to say?'. The accusation that autoethnography is uninteresting is one that is again voiced by Delamont (2009). For those who write autoethnography, this gross dismissal is unfair. For them, and for those who read autoethnography, it is also empirically without foundation. Autoethnographic writers testify to harrowing and cruel forms of social injustice of great cultural significance (see e.g. Holman Jones et al., 2013; Short et al., 2013; Turner et al., 2018). Public feedback to autoethnographers, including myself, suggests that readers are often comforted by autoethnographic accounts that speak helpfully and constructively to their own lives, and are useful in moving those lives forward. Moreover, in reality, readers are always likely to engage with autoethnography in a complex spectrum of ways (Grant, 2018a). You are one of them; what do you feel and think about autoethnography right now?

4　See Chapter Eleven.

References

Barthes, R. 1977. The Death of the Author. In Barthes, R., *Image-Music-Text: Essays Selected and Translated by Stephen Heath*. London: Fontana Press, 142–148.

Campell, E. 2017. 'Apparently Being a Self-Obsessed C★★t Is Now Academically Lauded': Experiencing Twitter Trolling of Autoethnographers. *Forum Qualitative Sozialforschung / Forum: Qualitative Social Research*, 18(3), Art16. http://dx.doi.org/10.17169/fqs-18.3.2819

Davies, B. and Harré, R. 1990. Positioning: The Discursive Production of Selves. *Journal for the Theory of Social Behaviour*, 20(1): 43–63.

Delamont, S. 2009. The Only Honest Thing: Autoethnography, Reflexivity and Small Crises in Fieldwork. *Ethnography and Education*, 4: 51–63.

Denzin, N.L. 2018. Autoethnography as Research Redux 1. In Turner, L., Short, N.P., Grant, A. and Adams, T.E. (eds.), *International Perspectives on Autoethnographic Research and Practice*. New York and Abingdon: Routledge, 35–54.

Denzin, N.K. and Lincoln, Y.S. 2000. Introduction. In Denzin, N.K. and Lincoln, Y.S. (eds.), *Handbook of Qualitative Research* (2nd ed.). Thousand Oaks, CA: SAGE, 1–29.

Diab, S. 2017. Writing Gown: The Challenges of Making a New Artwork about Sexism in Academia. In Cole, C. and Hassel, H. (eds.), *Surviving Sexism in Academia: Strategies for Feminist Leadership*. New York and London: Routledge, 89–97.

Frank, A.W. 2010. *Letting Stories Breathe: A Socio-narratology*. Chicago, IL: University of Chicago Press.

Grant, A. 2013. Writing, Teaching and Survival in Mental Health: A Discordant Quintet for One. In Short, N., Turner, L. and Grant, A. (eds.), *Contemporary British Autoethnography*. Rotterdam, Boston and Taipei: Sense Publishers, 33–48.

Grant, A. 2016a. Researching Outside the Box: Welcoming Innovative Qualitative Inquiry to Nurse Education Today. *Nurse Education Today*, 45: 55–56.

Grant, A. 2016b. Storying the World: A Posthumanist Critique of Phenomenological-Humanist Representational Practices in Mental Health Nurse Qualitative Inquiry. *Nursing Philosophy*, 17: 290–297.

Grant, A. 2016c. Living My Narrative: Storying Dishonesty and Deception in Mental Health Nursing. *Nursing Philosophy*, 17: 194–201.

Grant, A. 2017. Writing the Dead in Two Parts. In Sparkes, A. (ed.), *Auto/Biography Yearbook 2016*. Nottingham: Russell Press, 55–72.

Grant, A. Toilets Are the Proper Place for 'Outputs'! 2017. In Hayler, M. and J. Moriarty, J. (eds.), *Self-Narrative and Pedagogy: Stories of Experience within Teaching and Learning*. Rotterdam, Boston, MA and Taipei: Sense Publishers, 45–58.

Grant, A. Voice, Ethics, and the Best of Autoethnographic Intentions (or Writers, Readers, and the Spaces In-between). 2018a. In Turner, L., Short, N.P., Grant, A. and Adams, T.E. (eds.), *International Perspectives on Autoethnographic Research and Practice*. London and New York: Routledge, 107–122.

Grant, A. 2018b. Drinking to Relax: An Autoethnography of a Highland Family Viewed through a New Materialist Lens. In Sparkes, A. (ed.), *Auto/Biography Yearbook 2017*. Nottingham: Russell Press.

Grant, A. In press. Moving Around the Hyphens: A Critical Meta-autoethnographic Performance. In Williams, S. and Bull, P. (eds.), *Critical Mental Health Nursing*. Monmouth: PCCS Books.

Grant, A. and Zeeman, L. 2012. Whose Story Is It? An Autoethnography Concerning Narrative Identity. *The Qualitative Report (TQR)*, 17(72): 1–12.

Grant, A., Biley, F., Walker, H. and Leigh-Phippard, H. 2012. The Book, the Stories, the People: An Ongoing Dialogic Narrative Inquiry Study Combining a Practice

Development Project. Part 1: The Research Context. *Journal of Psychiatric and Mental Health Nursing*, 19: 844–851.

Grant, A., Short, N.P. and Turner, L. 2013. Introduction: Storying Life and Lives. In Short, N.P., Turner, L. and Grant, A. (eds.), *Contemporary British Autoethnography*. Rotterdam: Sense Publishers, 1–18.

Grant, A. and Leigh-Phippard, H. 2014. Troubling the Normative Mental Health Recovery Project: The Silent Resistance of a Disappearing Doctor. In Zeeman, L., Aranda, K. and Grant, A. (eds.), 2014. *Queering Health: Critical Challenges to Normative Health and Health-care*. Ross-on-Wye: PCCS Books, 100–115.

Grant, A., Leigh-Phippard, H. and Short, N.P. 2015. Re-storying Narrative Identity: A Dialogical Study of Mental Health Recovery and Survival. *Journal of Psychiatric and Mental Health Nursing*, 22: 278–286.

Holman Jones, S., Adams, T. and Ellis, C. 2013. Introduction: Coming to Know Auto-ethnography as More Than a Method. In Holman Jones, S., Adams, T.E. and Ellis, C. (eds.), *Handbook of Autoethnography*. Walnut Creek, CA: Left Coast Press, 17–48.

Klevan, T., Grant, A. and Karlsson, B. In press. Writing to Resist, Writing to Survive: Conversational Autoethnography, Mentoring, and the New Public Management Acad-emy. In Moriarty, J. (ed.), *Writing to Resist, Writing to Know: Autoethnographies from Higher Education*. London and New York: Routledge.

Klevan, T., Karlsson, B. and Grant, A. In review. The Color of Water and the Becoming of a Researcher – An Autoethnographically Inspired Journey. *The Qualitative Report (TQR)*.

Marcus, G. and Fischer, M., eds. 1986. *Anthropology as Cultural Critique*. Chicago, IL: Uni-versity of Chicago Press.

Minnich, E. 2017. *The Evil of Banality: On the Life and Death Importance of Thinking*. London: Rowman & Littlefield.

Moriarty, J. 2015. *Analytic Autoethnodrama: Autobiographed and Researched Experiences with Academic Writing*. Rotterdam, Boston and Taipei: Sense Publishers.

Pelias, R. 2011. Writing into Position: Strategies for Composition and Evaluation. In Denzin, N.K. and Lincoln, Y. (eds), *The SAGE Handbook of Qualitative Research* (4th ed.). London: SAGE, 666.

Richardson, L. 1997. *Fields of Play: Constructing an Academic Life*. New Brunswick, NJ: Rutgers University Press.

Richardson, L. 2001. Getting Personal: Writing-Stories. *International Journal of Qualitative Studies in Education*, 14(1): 33–38. doi:10.1080/09518390010007647

Short, N.P., Turner, L. and Grant, A., eds. 2013. *Contemporary British Autoethnography*. Rotterdam, Boston and Taipei: Sense Publishers.

Sorly, R., Karlsson, B. and Grant, A. In press. My Mother's Skull is Burning: A Story About Stories. In *Qualitative Inquiry*. Thousand Oaks, CA: SAGE.

Sparkes, A.C. 2002. *Telling Tales in Sport and Physical Activity: A Qualitative Journey*. Sta-ningley, Leeds: Human Kinetics.

Sparkes, A.C. 2018. Creating Criteria for Evaluating Autoethnography and the Pedagogical Potential of Lists. In Turner, L., Short, N.P., Grant, A. and T.E. Adams, T.E. (eds.), *International Perspectives on Autoethnographic Research and Practice*. New York and Abingdon: Routledge, 256–268.

Sparkes, A.C. In press. Autoethnography Comes of Age: Consequences, Comforts, and Concerns. In Beach, D., Bagley, C., Marques da Silva, S. (eds.), *Handbook of Ethnography of Education*. London: Wiley.

Turner, L., Short, N.P., Grant, A. and Adams, T.A., eds. 2018. *International Perspectives on Autoethnographic Research and Practice*. New York and Abingdon: Routledge.

Wright Mills, C. (1959/2000). *The Sociological Imagination*. Fortieth Anniversary Edition.New York: Oxford University Press.

Young, S. (Producer & Director). 2013. *It Started With a Murder* [Video file]. UK. Retrieved from https://vimeo.com/60178410

Young, S. (Producer & Director). 2015. *The Betrayal* [DCP]. UK. Retrieved from https://vimeo.com/126525542 *

10

POSTCRITICAL QUALITATIVE FEMINIST RESEARCH

Implications for participatory and narrative approaches

Kay Aranda

In this chapter I introduce and argue for a critical use of new materialist or material feminist theories and concepts to inform qualitative health research. New materialisms or material feminism in more-than-human worlds are being utilised to help rethink global health and care concerns. With social and health inequities still disproportionately affecting women around the world, and women's bodies remaining key sites of material, violent and symbolic struggles, especially in neoliberal times (Phipps, 2014), to think differently in order to act differently, using different research practices, is much needed.

To fully consider the philosophies, politics and practices of feminist research in a post materialist, qualitative era, we need to briefly revisit the histories of feminist research and the theories or philosophies and politics informing such practices. This reacquaintance with previous histories is also important for understanding the ongoing critical interrogations of feminist theory, politics and research requires, including use of new materialisms and material feminism. Any feminist research is best understood as informed by diverse understandings of feminisms, with their range of inspiration from philosophies, theories, activism and research practices, as global networks of emerging, entangled, relational knowledges and politics, concerned with and connected to ethical practices that are historically contingent or situated. Given this complexity and diversity of thought, any discussion of feminist research moves beyond naive stereotypes or readings, refuses asserting self-evident truths and instead offers a critical engagement as well as interrogation with feminist theory, politics and research. This suggests a more modest set of claims in order to explore, confront, expand, extend and revise understandings of our contemporary shared worlds.

Feminist philosophies, theories and politics

Feminist theories, philosophies, politics and practices continue to ask why women, as well as others who are marginal, misrecognized or invisible, continue to experience disproportionate levels of inequalities and precarity (Butler, 2004a). There is therefore an explicit commitment to social justice and social change. This is not theorising or research generating abstract knowledge, but rather an explicit intent for research to be applied to further progressive transformative social change. In this sense, all feminist research is explicitly critical and political (Harding, 2004; Letherby, 2003; Hesse-Biber, 2014). One of feminisms' greatest contribution has been a commitment to interrogation, challenging the norms of objectivity of western scientific research to reveal the partiality of all knowledge making. The gendered or masculine values and patriarchal interests represented in such claims exposed the myopic, androcentric nature of much western theorising. This generated an invisibility and marginalisation of women and their concerns and issues as trivial, not worthy of consideration or of little practical importance or theoretical interest (Tong, 2013). To insist on recognition of the political, gendered historical processes in all knowledge production was to argue that what passed as neutral and unbiased was in fact androcentric, phallocentric and ethnocentric (Harding, 2004). The claims for a view from nowhere was instead a view from somewhere (Tong, 2013).

From the canon of feminist theories, be that liberal, radical, Marxist, socialist, Black, or standpoint, psychoanalytical to queer, postcolonial and poststructural feminism, a significant body of research documents women's health and illness and their lived experiences, giving voice, making visible, and/or celebrating particular and specific knowledges and viewpoints (Letherby, 2003; Harding, 2004). Many examples exist, from research revealing the medicalisation of birth, of women's health and illness but especially their bodies (Tong, 2013; Annandale, 2009; Annandale & Hunt, 2000), to documenting women's invisibility in accounts of heart disease, or in discriminatory experiences of mental health and primary care (Roberts, 1992; Doyal, 1995). Feminist research exposed the systemic nature of gender relations governing healthcare systems, producing, maintaining and reproducing gender relations through organizational practices, producing workplace disadvantage and discrimination (Kuhlmann & Annandale, 2012). Further analyses revealed how deeply embedded androcentrism was together with systemic racism, ageism, ableism and heterosexism in healthcare. This research challenged what mattered or counted in terms of health research, expanding these concerns to include domestic life, housework, sexuality and reproduction (Kuhlmann & Annandale, 2012).

In poststructural or postcolonial feminism ontological and epistemological assumptions start with notions of reality or realities as continuously emergent effects of dominant discursive practices that are normatively gendered, classed and racialised. The aim therefore is to identify meanings, metaphors, images, stories or statements that produce these specific versions of events, while excluding others.

This is a position that rejects modernity's stories of progress of grand narratives of progress or civilization through science and the sovereignty of the subject as the source of authoritative knowledge. Instead historically and culturally variable ways of knowledge coming together with power circulate to produce truths that are never fixed, but contingent, situated, and relational but that have damaging material effects. Using Foucauldian notions of power as dispersed /resistance/ productive not merely repressive, discourses operate with notions of language as performative, actively constructing or inscribing, governing and disciplining identities or subject position of healthcare (Cheek, 2000; Aranda, 2006).

Despite these informative studies, feminist theory informed research remains either invisible or a minority interest in much health-related research (Lupton, 2019; Broom, 2014). Reasons for this are difficult to ascertain but the difficult contexts feminism now operates in with intensified neoliberalism resulting in governments giving priority to economic growth, low taxes, freedom and individual personal choice or restating traditional values, means feminism with logics of seeking collective mobilization or solidarity for social justice stand in opposition to and conflict with neoconservative and neoliberal rationalities (Fraser, 2008, 2013; Walby, 2011; Phipps, 2014). Moreover, the very term feminism continues to have negative connotations of separatism or extremism for some, or more recently, of being considered irrelevant and redundant give neoliberal notions of individual choice and personal lived experience so highly central and valued in western healthcare (Broom, 2014). Moreover, feminism has been thought to have lost its purpose, even colluding with neoliberal ideologies and imperatives in celebrating individual agency or power (Gill & Orgad, 2015). Additionally, having seemed more interested in abstract theorising than conducting research into material issues still impacting upon women's lives (Einstein & Shildrick, 2009), feminists are accused of deserting politics, ignoring struggles for the radical redistribution of resources in the pursuit of social justice and progressive change (Fraser, 2013). Finally, as a modern social movement driven by gender inequality and exclusion within modern liberal democratic states, most feminisms, even poststructural feminism, retain an enlightenment legacy of humanism that is now under sustained critique (Andrews & Duff, 2019). This inheritance is to be found in various ways in current feminist research; from notions of valuing the human subject, how they create, understand and experience or give meanings to health and illness, or in the essentialist belief of a shared nature or biology, or sharing common experiences of oppression, to including the possibility of identifying universal causes of women's subordination. Although these assumptions were seriously challenged with the rise of identity politics and a politics of difference and then intersectional feminisms, with respective significant critiques from postcolonial, Black critical, transnational and indigenous feminist theorising, the initial inadequate response of feminism to difference furthered the ontological and epistemological as well as political crisis (Mohanty, 1988; Hill Collins, 2000; hooks, 1982; Falcón, 2016). With the arrival of poststructural theorising within feminism, critical scrutiny and suspicion of all theorising and research practices evolved. In recognising these limits and critiques, feminist theory, politics and research has sought to readdress these harms and exclusions. The notable "silent privileging of the Northern white, middle class, heterosexual and able-bodied subject of some feminist theorising" (Ryan-Flood & Gill, 2010, p. 4) led to extensive scrutiny over voice and representation being complicit with, and actively constituting 'the Other' in research. Further critical revisions and reflexivity were needed. This is evident in responses to postcolonial feminist arguments for decolonizing research methodologies (Smith, 2012) and in developing more inclusive, non-additive accounts of difference, working with concepts of intersectionality through empirical research (Crenshaw, 1991; Hankivsky 2011, 2012). Contemporary feminist research therefore seeks to question naive, romantic notions of voice or experience, revealing instead the inherent power relations or social constructionist nature of such, as well as the assumption of a transcendental viewpoint or view from nowhere with a view of all knowledge, including feminisms' own, as contingent, perspectival and partial (Jackson & Mazzei, 2012; Haraway, 1988).

Feminist research practices

Given the aforementioned multiplicity of theories and critiques it remains useful to note what makes feminist research distinctive. Research can be said to be feminist when it is grounded in aforementioned theoretical traditions privileging gendered processes, relations and structures as well as issues, voices and experiences of what initially became synonymous with women's issues or lived experiences. This was and often remains research on, for and about women (Hesse-Biber, 2014). Though it is research which places gender as the key category at the centre of inquiry (Hesse-Biber, 2012, 2014; Letherby, 2003). As such, more recent focus is on the concept of gender as a lived relation operating in both visible and invisible ways across spheres considered public and private, that is both felt to be individual and personal but also socially derived and systemic, even operating as a pervasive, organizing mechanism in society, arranging and influencing lives, opportunities and experiences (Springer, Hankivsky, & Bates, 2012).

To undertake feminist research then is to gain insights into the gendered nature of social life and existence. Placing gender as a principle at the centre of inquiry is to assume that gender profoundly shapes and mediates the very condition of our lives. More recently, what constitutes the category of gender and/or woman has been the source of further controversy and remains very much a part of academic as well as public debate and discussion (Cooper, 2019). These discussions, over who gets to be counted as a woman, or how expansive or redundant a binary concept of gender is, further shows the politics or power of language and its material effects. This conceptual binary struggle will no doubt impact on future feminist research in challenging and troubling key assumptions and ideas underpinning our notions of woman and gender (Cooper, 2019).

Feminist research additionally seeks to trouble or deconstruct traditional commitments to truth, objectivity and neutrality. As plural and diverse perspectives in

Postcritical qualitative feminist research **181**

research, feminists use a multiplicity of method but have in common a view of knowledge creation as partial or perspectival (Hekman, 1990). A further defining characteristic of feminist research is the concept of praxis. This understanding of the practices of research and its relationship to theory is conceived as a dialectical, reciprocal, often collaborative form of knowledge production (Lather 1991, 2015, 2016). This is a research practice which pays attention to the dynamics of power and authority between researcher and participant, usually addressed through practices of reflexivity (Hesse-Biber, 2014). These practices of praxis and reflexivity are said to offer ways of being accountable for these dimensions of power and authority and their effects. Feminist research as such wishes to generate morally accountable understandings and relevant knowledge aiming to drive or ensure progressive or transformative socio-political change.

Definitions of methodology as a theoretical and conceptual framework with which research proceeds (Harding, 2004), is a useful reminder of the ways theory always connects to methodology. So whilst feminist methodology, informed by feminist theories and concepts, frames the research, in the design of any given project, there are no one set of methods deemed to be feminist (Letherby, 2003; Ramazanoglu & Holland, 2002). Feminist make full use of quantitative, mixed methods as well as qualitative approaches, including creative and arts-based methods (Hesse-Biber, 2012; Hesse Biber & Leavy, 2008; Reinharz, 1992).

The profound scrutiny and interrogation of feminisms politics and theories has led to diversification of approaches and experimenting with novel methods to break away from protocol or rule driven approaches of only one right linear way to conduct research, often a mimesis of the scientific approach to knowledge. There is now a complex ecology, with inventing, innovating practices being demanded (Lather & St. Pierre, 2013). Yet what this means practically for qualitative health research is less than clear at present. Even when acknowledging the limits to essentialist concepts of woman, and attempting to be premised on diverse concepts of woman, experience or subjectivity, these new materialist approaches of the more than human world disrupt understandings of core taken for granted assumptions and concepts at the heart of qualitative health research such as agency, the authority of human experience or divides between subject and object or nature and the social world. For conventional qualitative health research methodologies or inquiries, such as narrative or participatory research, the full implications of these new theories are less clear.

The narrative turn is part of a larger epistemic turn to language in history, anthropology, psychology, sociology, cultural studies and humanities. Blurring boundaries between humanities and science, narrative research combines art and science as it includes a scientific process but also a creative component that generates an effect (Freshwater & Holloway, 2007). Like much interpretative and poststructural qualitative research assumes, no two stories will be similar. If a story is recreated or retold it will differ from the original. Narratives are culturally, contextually and time specific.

Participatory research starts from an explicit commitment to addressing power relations in knowledge production. Using an asset or strengths-based approach, this research aims to democratize research, forming partnerships with communities based on radically different values to traditional expert led research. This research is driven by values of inclusion, collaboration, sharing power, developing trust, often work from the ground up, tackling issues that matter most to local people or non-academic stakeholders (Leavy, 2017; Brinton Lykes & Crosby, 2014). These approaches emerge from the valuing of experiential knowledge and a transformative social justice paradigm, with desires for more action orientated research using inclusive, emancipatory methods such as photovoice (Wang, 1999; Mertens, 2007; Palmer et al., 2018).

Both narrative and participatory research are far from uniform methodologies, operating in diverse ways and informed by different interdisciplinary theories and political intents (Andrews, Squire, & Tamboukou, 2008; Hesse-Biber, 2012). However, the starting point for most narrative and participatory research remains with the sovereignty of the individual autonomous person or centrality of human experience in understanding phenomena, and with concepts of power as possessive, or most often with unproblematic notions of experience, voice, or subjectivity as cognitive or emotional affective properties of human subjects alone. The world outside of the human subject is conceived as secondary in causes, influence, or factors; and as instrumental to any given subject's use. A closer alignment to new materialist feminist theories can be found in those narrative and participatory approaches drawing on poststructural theories.

Poststructural accounts of narratives understand language as a form of doing, which is unstable and complex and importantly, with meanings not self-evidently driven by human intent or deliberation (Tamboukou, 2008). Narratives instead reflect larger discourses of meaning, power and social norms, constructing particular versions of the world that shape human thought and experience. So that telling and re-telling stories drawing on dominant discourses of femininity, motherhood, of home or work, health and wellbeing, serve to create a sense of self and plural identity positions (Woodiwiss, Smith, & Lockwood, 2017; Burr, 2003). Yet how these dominant discourses and meanings emerge or are shaped or entangled with the material world is overlooked or ignored. Even when identity is considered socially constructed and constituted through the stories we tell or broader discourses, it remains social rather than natural worlds that are cited as sources of origin or influence.

Feminist participatory research seeks to pursue more democratic or egalitarian ways of creating or coproducing knowledge and conducting research. These approaches have the potential to democratize and decolonize research practices and knowledge. However, in exploring how power circulates in such methodologies and practices, Janes (2016) suggests these intents and potentials may be otherwise. Using postcolonial theories as a productive lens, she seeks to trouble the discursive claims, often unwarranted or critically examined, of giving voice, or of equality in the material practices, subject positions and spaces of collaborative knowledge work. Rather, she reveals the means by which academic epistemic power and position remains privileged and is sustained.

Materialist feminist philosophies, theories and research

Poststructural feminism, together with other postfeminist research drawing on queer or postcolonial theories, contribute much that is valuable in deconstructing core binaries, concepts or norms. However, in these analyses, language, rather than matter or material, still remained privileged, words were felt to have too much say (Butler, 1990; Barad, 2007). The more recent turn to matter evident in material feminism or new materialisms is a collective term for the turn to matter in contemporary thought that seeks to revise this privileging of words over materials. It includes material feminisms and other similar work, building on a posthuman thought to explore the social world and the active role of matter and materials.

Most new materialist writing acknowledges or actively draws on feminist scholars such as Barad (2007), Alaimo and Hekman (2008), Haraway (2008), Bennett (2010), Coole and Frost (2010) and Braidotti (2013), though not all materialist theories arise from feminist concerns. This move towards understandings of the agency or liveliness of matter and its disruption of the subject/object binary can be seen previously in Bruno Latour's (2007) work, and his account of reassembling the social world where materials are conceived as actants: this means objects, technology, or things have agency; or in the philosophies of Delueze and Guattari (2004), proposing nomadic or rhizomic knowledges and assemblages. A theoretical move towards notions of materials as performative, as doing something beyond human intention or will, is similarly present in recent epistemic turns to practice in posthuman practice-based theorising. In practice theory, health is reconceived not as individual behaviours but as sets of practices, generating revised notions of cause, effect, behaviour or change (Hui, Schatzki, & Shove, 2017; Aranda & Hart, 2014, 2015; Cohn, 2014)

Cutting across the dualisms of research e.g. realism or constructionism, postitivism or interpretivism, qualitative or quantitative, objective or subjective, these posthuman theories present a radical shift in understandings of the subject/object nature/culture dualism. A number of key feminist authors are influential in this tradition including Karen Barad, Jane Bennett, Rosi Braditotti and Donna Haraway. These theories inform and reshape qualitative research methodologies by de-privileging human agency to focus instead on how the world is configured or made up of assemblages of animate and inanimate subjects/objects, the more than human world, that together, in intra-action, produce the messy realities we recognise as our world. As Donna Haraway (2008) argues, as companion species, humans are continually 'becoming with' microbes, other animals, technologies, and spaces.

This challenges the divide or binary common in public health or the social sciences and qualitative research, between either nature or culture or the physical or social environment. For healthcare or public health, these new materialist theories point to the pertinence of our entanglement with the more than human world, a natureculture, and knowledge practices like research premised upon an ontoepistemology (Barad, 2007). What has been less clear are the implications both for research methodologies and methods from this type of thinking.

The full implications of these theories for qualitative health research are still relatively new. However, such theories suggest reimagining the whole endeavour; seeing practices, philosophies and politics of research as research assemblages, configured, aligning and reconfiguring; practices that unfold or fold back (Fox & Alldred, 2017). In questioning the assumed human capacity to produce research knowledge as always from the point of view of the researcher, new materialism theories challenge the anthropocentric privileging of human cognitive processes. Instead, objects, bodies and space and gender and embodied practices of mattering become the focus for qualitative health research (Andrews & Duff, 2019; Lupton, 2019; Taylor & Hughes, 2016).

Key assumptions include:

- Objects, bodies and space as vital materialities possess dynamic agency
- Agency is distributed not possessed
- Material cultures are active and constitutive in processes that recreate gender inequalities
- Space is not simply a physical container for human action, space, place, environment and context entangled with human and non-human in the more than human world
- Objects and things are not inert, fixed or passive matter awaiting 'use' by human intervention
- Body is not a mere corporeal vehicle to be moved by the mind
- Health is a continuously emergent assemblage of bodies, subjectivities, agencies, objects, technologies, affect, attachments and desires.
- A diffractive methodology encourages new ways of thinking about and relating to data and meaning-making
- Offers a critical disruptive practice which pays attention to what we don't normally see, to what is excluded, brings context to the fore.
- Urges commitment to understanding the more than human world and which differences matter, how they matter, and for whom.

New materialist ontology is not necessarily anti-binaries, Lather (2016) suggests, but rather there is an interest in how binaries come undone or falter and dissolve in breaking through the mind/matter/culture nature divides and other dominant dualisms of structure/agency or reason/emotion and human and nonhuman. A theory of posthuman agency means action, free will or behaviour or intent is not located in humans and their bodies, but is to be found instead in relational networks of materials, meanings, competencies and affects. Matter is no longer now simply the background for human activity, the material world is instead conceptualised as multiple nonhuman, as well as human, sources of agency with capacities to affect.

The question over what is new exactly is a reminder of previous research accounts of materialism to be found in studies of living conditions i.e. reproduction, roles and labour in family, workplace, inequalities or divisions. This materialism, often of Marxism, is evident in but differentiated from the new materialism of recent feminist theorising (Jaggar, 2015). Moreover, statements of newness might be Eurocentric in depicting concerns of white Western ontology in research, troubled by these new theories, when indigenous knowledges have always considered the more than human world in their accounts of the life (Smith, 2012). What is different from previous western notions of material or matter is that matter, biology, bodies, technology, objects are no longer static but considered vital, agentic, even perverse, and beyond human control or use. Such thinking decentres humans as the source of knowledge or as the drivers of change. Instead there is a focus on the more than human world and a notion of matter as materialising through relationality, processes and becoming. This is a non-essentialist account, with states of being as fluid, unfolding, not fixed, enduring or static. In decentring the human subject, technologies and objects, for example, come to the fore and have been shown to actively shape understandings, actions, identities and subjectivities. This is a flatter ontology of assemblages or practices producing, material capacities from this nexus of human and nonhuman relations.

Research interest and focus is over engagements/entanglements with matter, and how discourse and matter intra-act and are mutually constituted in knowing (Jackson & Mazzei, 2012). These theories acknowledge the closeness of non-human worlds to human concerns in health and illness. Producing new accounts of theory–practice relations, these accounts de-centre human activity, not just by adding in materiality, they pull context to the fore as more than just a backdrop to the drama of human life or human agency or cognition. This makes visible the often invisible and reworks binaries of subject–object and nature–culture. However, what this means for research in terms of methodology or method is not yet fully worked out but many are using such insights to develop different understanding of health, illness and care which I discuss next.

Material feminism and more-than-human-world research

Drawing on these understandings means the concern in research is not just with human bodies or objects or things, or social institutions, but with the practices or capacities for action, interaction, and the feeling and desire produced in and through networks of practices or assemblages. It is this landscape of dynamic configurations, and reconfigurations, entanglements, relationalities and re-articulations that become the units of analysis. The discursive material practices that enact flows of agency are what constitutes the ongoing reconfiguration of the world (Barad, 2007). Neither discourse or matter has privilege in these theories so knowledge or being is not to be prioritized. This a flatter ontology or an entangled notion of ontology and epistemology, indicated in the Baradian term ontoepistemology. Postconventional understandings of human agency the division between agency and structure disappears as relations in the assemblage cut across the material, culture dualism and across micro, mess and macro levels of analysis as materiality is dynamic and is a becoming rather than being.

The full implications of these ideas for health sciences theories and research suggest a radical, thorough, ongoing interrogation of all core assumptions and key concepts in order to reimagine the practices of research (Fox & Alldred, 2017). The shift towards a materialist form of social inquiry dissolves the dualism between realist and constructionist accounts of the world and focuses instead on a revised, flatter ontology, or the kind of things that exist in the world, including humans. This ontological shift is away from essences and being, to processes and becoming, or a concern with what matter does.

Revised methodologies and tools of inquiry aim to map this dynamic world of differential flows, energies, affect and desires as the assemblages that emerge become the phenomena to be understood. What this might look like for critical health-related empirical research is beginning to emerge (Fox & Alldred, 2017; Lather & St. Pierre, 2013; Lather, 2016). In de-privileging human agency the focus becomes instead on how the world is configured or made up of assemblages of animate and inanimate subjects/objects, that together in intra-action produce the messy realities we recognise as our world. In questioning the anthropocentric privileging of human cognitive processes, new materialist ontology take agency, action, free will or behaviour or intent not to be only located in humans or their bodies. Instead, agency is to be found in relational networks of materials, meanings, competencies and affects. This approach profoundly challenges the implicit inherent representational claims of change, agency or structure and seeks instead to pay attention to the way entities like health, illness, care or inequality, as practices, are co-constitutive of the realities they enact or bring into being. This approach to knowledge for example critiques biomedical individualised accounts of illness, with research on depression or recovery, seeking instead to identify the enabling and impeding dimensions of place or emplacement that at the same time are affective, gendered, social and material (Fullagar & O'Brien, 2010; Fullagar, 2017).

These postconventional understandings of human agency are suggesting radically different accounts of action or change, or of the ways in which life, history, or societies unfold. Research units of analysis shift from the subject or agent to assemblages or practices, and a concern not necessarily with human bodies, or objects, or things, or social institutions, but with the practices or capacities for action, interaction, and the feeling and desire produced in and through these networks, practices or assemblages (Fox & Alldred, 2017). Thus, divisions between agency and structure disappear as relations in the assemblage cut across the material or nature/culture dualism and across micro-, mess- and macro-levels of analysis. These assemblages of relations develop in unpredictable ways, creating networks of habitual and non-habitual connections that any empirical research would seek to analyse and understand (Fox & Alldred, 2017).

Material feminisms and critical qualitative health research examples

Increasing use of new materialist and material feminisms theories now exist to explore health, illness and care research. Many studies speculate and propose the potential and new insights to be gained in for example studying or understanding eating disorders, masculinity or sexuality, or in considering the visceral nature of birth, as assemblages of sociomaterial embodied relations (Fox & Alldred, 2017; Lupton & Schmied 2012). Public health concerns inevitably involve bodies and nowhere is this notion of the body more deeply implicated than in the global debates over obesity. Drawing on the turn to matter, philosopher Jane Bennett (2010) questions what happens to public health when we view food and eating practices through these new materialist lenses. Eating would become an assemblage made up of forces, desires, of human and nonhuman entities that are beyond individual control. She considers what happens when we understand eating and food relations where matter, like food, has a vitality that defies human intent. For Bennett (2010) vitality refers to the capacity of things to hinder or undermine the will of humans and that matter or things have propensities or tendencies of their own. Similarly, she argues understandings would change if food or eating practices are not simply assume or consider food as a mere resource, commodity or instrument, but as an actant. She draws on Actor Network Theory and Latour's (2007) understanding of things as a source of action; meaning food does things; it produces effects. This suggests a more distributed agency with human and nonhuman entities being on a less vertical plane; a flatter ontology (Bennett, 2010) than in the ontology of realist and constructionist humanism.

She asks what happens to an understanding of public health when we view eating as an assemblage of forces, desires, of human and nonhuman entities rather than entirely under individual control. She argues for conceptions of food as an actant, within a particular agentic assemblage - often nonlinear, producing transforming effects inside the body and mind seen in changes in emotions or affect, in biochemistry, metabolism, and of course outside size, shape, and self and other response. She states:

> The idea of bodies as changing over time, shedding, ageing, ingesting and excreting food water gases microorganisms – and not fixed or static, with permeable boundaries ingesting excreting, reshaping, relating to technologies not ending or beginning – this views of the human body as profoundly connected nature in everyday life revealed in assemblages troubles dominant notions of the independent subject that continue to pervade health and care practices.
>
> *(Bennett, 2010, p. x)*

This type of theorisation seriously challenges dominant individualised shame and blame discourses of biomedical accounts of obesity. The theoretical and analytical demand is for a full account of resources and materials involved in such

188 Kay Aranda

phenomena; features long argued to be conveniently overlooked in much inequalities research (Bambra et al., 2011). Materialist feminist accounts offer deeper understandings of how socially, culturally and materially the phenomena of inequalities, of obesity and health, emerge or materialise as a product of human and nonhuman relations (Warin, 2014).

In sports and health sciences, the importance of fully understanding gendered mental health and recovery requires studies of both human and nonhuman relations (Fullagar, 2017; Fullagar & O'Brien, 2010); and in policy studies, scholars have shown how ethical imperatives of care come to matter in and through policy (Gill, Singleton, & Waterton, 2017), or how these theories expose relations of humans to nonhumans, objects, materials, environments, technologies in matters of care in more than human worlds (Puig de la Bellacasa, 2017). Other public health scholars have similarly explored the active materiality of environments or technologies involved in constructing, enabling or shaping the so called healthy subject or subjectivities (Maller, 2015; Maller & Strengers, 2019), as well as the role of materials in reconceptualised notions of resilience as critical, resistive, politicised socio–material practices, and how these relate to tackling inequalities (Aranda & Hart, 2014).

Research questions, methodologies and methods and analysis

Materialist methodologies suggested by Fox and Alldred (2017) propose an ontological orientation towards matter as opposed to texts or structures; a concern with what matter does, not what it is; a post-anthropocentric focus on capacity of all matter to affect; recognition that thoughts, memories, desires and emotions have material effects; power and resistance operates at the local level of action and events – rather than top down; changes how we think or claim change occurs (Aranda, 2018). Given this, research becomes conceived as an assemblage. As sets of performative practices or assemblages of actors, tools, technologies, emotions, desires, motivations, meanings, skills, knowledge, bodies, memories, place or history, research works with understandings of agency as distributed. Action, free will or experience, behaviour or intent is not located in humans and their bodies but is to be found instead in relational networks of materials, meanings, competencies and affects (Fox & Alldred, 2014).

More recently, Lupton (2019) has argued more specifically for inspiration from these new materialist, material feminist theories of the more than human world offer for health related research. Using her own empirical research in digital health technologies designed to monitor and promote health, she explores this potential. She aims to address the 'vagueness or even mystique' around how to do applied feminist material research. Arguing for these novel ways for analysing human subjectivities, embodiment, agency and power relations in a more than human world (Lupton 2019, p. 1), she documents her approach to show how these theories impact on research questions, bring into view different research materials and produce fresh insights.

Lupton (2019) shows how different questions become possible as these are inquiries over the key human and nonhuman practices, imaginaries, assumptions and discourses operating across different sites and spaces relating to health. She asks how health, care and illness are configured and enacted; or what can human bodies do when coming together with things and places? As importantly, these theories enable questions about the potentials for thinking or doing otherwise. In her research with health technologies, these theories help identify the micropolitical dimensions of people's engagements with things, spaces, and places. This allows for attending to the complexities and details of how people come together with healthcare, with other practitioners and the roles of politics, technologies or objects in places so deepening understandings of these enactments (Lupton 2019, p. 5). In asking what bodies can do when they assemble with nonhumans, fresh insights concerning agential capacities, affective forces and relational connections. Her research insights include confirming the significance of biographical experiences, or relational connections to desires for health, fitness, enjoyment of nature and movement through exercise. She concludes instead of research method, qualitative health researchers using these theories should consider an approach of 'lively assemblages of thinking and doing' for how to go about research (Lupton, 2019, p. 10).

Critical physiotherapists draw upon new materialist ideas to further these detailed micro-political accounts. Conceiving of technology as part of more or less stable assemblages of bodies, things and spaces that have the capacities to enable or constrain, Gibson et al. (2016) explore the experiences of young people with disabilities. Using these theories decentres the autonomous subject of western neoliberal healthcare to allow analysis of the interactions between humans and nonhuman entities, but without privileging one over the other. This they suggest creates a space to interrogate how people's abilities/inabilities are produced – and how different subjects are enacted through various configurations of elements (Gibson et al., 2016). In challenging biomedical accounts these theories offer opportunities for changes in rehabilitation practices, through fine-grained analysis of socio-technical interactions (Gibson et al., 2016, p. 4).

A further health related example of the importance of full context and materials can be found in Mol's (2008) work on competing logics of choice and care in healthcare systems. Using these theoretical frames, the whole context comes to the fore in order to follow the sociomaterial orderings or configurations of meanings and matter that comprise practices of logics of choice and care. Interviews were not about asking people about their opinions but about the events and activities they were involved in. In this way, patients and staff offered knowledge about the treatment involved in living a life with diabetes. Mol separates out good care from messy practices. She argues that gathering knowledge is not matter of providing better maps of reality but of crafting more bearable ways of living with or in reality (Mol 2008, p. 53).

Although not health related research, in thinking with theory in qualitative research, Jackson and Mazzei (2012) draw upon Barad to analysing data using 'diffraction' from these new materialist perspectives. They argue diffraction removes us from habitual or normative readings of data or texts, in similar ways to a discursive approach, but here discourse is more than language. Meaning is always already material, but so too is the material world always already discursively constituted. This mutuality of constitution is similarly evident Barad's concept of intra-action. The term inter-action concerns two separate bodies or entities, whereas for Barad the term intra-action captures the entanglement of relations with both the dynamic nature of material and meaning. For example, the body in healthcare is frequently conceived as produced by and entangled in sociomaterial or affective relations that constitute embodiment (Draper, 2014; Aranda, 2018).

In new materialist theories bodies are understood as temporal and emplaced, emerging from and entangled in both material and discursive relations. A further Baradian term they draw on is agential realism. This concept aims to more adequately capture the dynamic distributed properties of agency. Agency becomes ascribed not only to humans, but to the nonhuman, the material and discursive, natural and cultural worlds and other sociomaterial practices (Barad, 2007). Agency is then not an attribute or property of anything or subject. This is the landscape for research; of dynamic configurations, and reconfigurations, entanglements and relationalities and re-articulations that become the units of analysis, not through words, but in the discursive material practices that enact this flow of agency. There are no individual effects of either discourse or matter, they are intertwined and together constitute the intra-action that is agency in the world.

These theories mean more than inserting the material into the data or meaning making in a qualitative study (Jackson & Mazzei, 2012). This theoretical frame shifts the focus from the way individuals make choices or acting, to how forces of material conditions, such as location or size of home or an office and the materiality of bodies work together. This is a movement from 'what is told' to 'what is produced'. This is inclusive of non-human and human bodies, identities or subjectivities and things seen in artefacts such as furniture, rooms, books, space and clothes (Jackson & Mazzei, 2012).

Limits to material feminisms and feminist research

While the potentials of these ways of thinking suggest new insights of our complex, entangled lives with the more than human world, there are recognised struggles to envisage this more pragmatically, and both point to the dangers or effort it takes to move beyond liberal humanist qualitative methodologies (St. Pierre, 2015; Lather, 2015). For St. Pierre, qualitative researchers have already failed to fully realise the radical posthuman moment or turn of poststructuralism, merely instead inserting traditional methods into a study using theoretical ideas that in the end retained a lurking humanism. She advocates new practices for research and much of these include reading, in depth, for a considerable period to immerse researchers into the often abstract, complex, difficult reads of the seminal authors they wish their work to be informed by. For Lather, the ethico-ontoepistemological entanglements similarly imply radical departure or new practices of research should not merely insert theory into what are humanist methods of interviews for example. She argues for reading to be one the practices that should be embedded in this ontological turn, or this post posthuman way of conceiving the world; what then emerges is yet to be seen.

There also remains a question over what is exactly new about these theories. Previous accounts of materialism are to be found in studies of living conditions i.e. reproduction, roles and labour in family, workplace, inequalities or divisions in political economy approached to health and illness or Marxist materialism. Although importantly what differentiates new materialism of recent feminist theorising from these previous accounts is the agentic, relational and affective understandings of matter together with meaning. Previous western notions of material or matter is here that matter, biology, bodies, technology, objects are no longer static but considered vital, agentic, even perverse, and beyond human control or use, always entangled and emergent. Such thinking decentres humans as the source of knowledge or as the drivers of change (Jaggar, 2015). Moreover, statements of newness suggest a deep eurocentrism in depicting concerns of white Western ontology in research whereas other indigenous knowledges have always considered the more than human world (Smith, 2012).

Conclusion

Material feminisms offer qualitative health researchers non essentialist accounts with potentials for detailed complex studies reasserting the importance of materials as resources and in exploring the relational, connected and agentic ways health, illness or care come to materialise, are configured and reconfigured as states of being as fluid, unfolding, not fixed, enduring or static. In decentring the human subject, other research materials and matters come to the fore, such as connections or entanglements with technologies and objects, which actively shape understandings, actions, identities and subjectivities. This flatter ontology of assemblages or practices producing, material capacities from this nexus of human and nonhuman relations allows researchers to focus on the more than human world materialising through relationality, processes and becoming. This allows different questions to be raised with different insights produced. Material feminist philosophies, politics generate sets of research practices revealing overlooked materials as resources, be they bodies, tools and/or technologies, which materialise together to deepen our understandings of complex worlds in which health and care unfold. Furthermore, these developments, far from being a threat to feminist research, provide a critical, urgent impetus to political arguments for resources and the valuing of often misrecognised or invisible practices of health and care.

References

Alaimo, S. and Hekman, S. (eds.) (2008) *Material Feminisms*. Bloomington: Indiana University Press.

Andrews, G. and Duff, C. (2019) 'Matter beginning to matter: on posthumanist understandings of the vital emergence of health', *Social Science & Medicine*, 226, 123–134.

Andrews, M., Squire, C. and Tamboukou, M. (2008) *Doing Narrative Research*. London: Sage.

Annandale, E. (2009) *Women's Health and Social Change*. London: Routledge.

Annandale, E. and Hunt, K. (2000) *Gender Inequalities in Health*. Buckingham: Open University Press.

Aranda, K. (2006) 'Postmodern feminist perspectives and nursing research: a passionately interested form of inquiry', *Nursing Inquiry*, 13(2), 135–143.

Aranda, K. (2018) *Feminist Theories and Concepts in Healthcare: An Introduction for Qualitative Research*. London: Palgrave Macmillan.

Aranda, K. and Hart, A. (2014) 'Resilient moves: tinkering with practice theory to generate new ways of thinking about using resilience', *Health*, 19(4), 355–371.

Aranda, K. and Hart, A. (2015) 'Developing resilience and practice theory', *Primary Health Care: The RCN Community Nursing Journal*, 25(10), 18–25.

Bambra, C., Smith, K. E., Garthwaite, K., Joyce, K. E. and Hunter, D. J. (2011) 'A labour of Sisyphus? Public policy and health inequalities research from the Black and Acheson Reports to the Marmot Review', *Journal of Epidemiology and Community Health*, 65(5), 399–406.

Barad, K. (2007) *Meeting the Universe Halfway: Quantum Physics and the Entanglement of Matter and Meaning*. Durham, NC and London: Duke University Press.

Bennett, J. (2010) *Vibrant Matter: A Political Ecology of Things*. London: Duke University Press.

Braidotti, R. (2013) *The Posthuman*. Cambridge: Polity.

Brinton Lykes, M. and Crosby, A. (2014) 'Feminist practice of action and community research'. In Hesse-Biber, S. N. (ed.), *Feminist Research Practice: A Primer*. London: SAGE, pp. 145–181.

Broom, D. (2014) 'Feminism in the social sciences of health and illness', *Australian Feminist Studies*, 29(80), 171–179.

Burr, V. (2003) *An Introduction to Social Constructionism* (2nd ed.). London: Routledge.

Butler, J. (2004a) *Precarious Life: The Powers of Mourning and Violence*. London: Verso.

Butler, J. (2004b) *Undoing Gender*. London: Routledge.

Butler, J. (1990) *Gender Trouble: Feminism and the Subversion of Identity*. London: Routledge.

Cheek, J. (2000) *Postmodern and Poststructural Approaches to Nursing Research*. London: SAGE.

Cohn, S. (ed.) (2014) *Health Behaviours to Health Practices*. Oxford: Blackwell.

Coole, D. and Frost, S. (eds.) (2010) *New Materialisms: Ontology, Agency, and Politics*. Durham, NC and London: Duke University Press.

Cooper, D. (2019) 'A very binary drama: the conceptual struggle for gender's future', *feminists@law*, 9(1), 1–36.

Crenshaw, K. (1991) 'Mapping the margins: intersectionality, identity politics, and violence against women of color', *Stanford Review*, 43(6), 1241–1299.

Deleuze, G. and Guattari, F. (2004) *A Thousand Plateaus: Capitalism and Schizophrenia*. London: Continuum.

Doyal, L. (1995) *What Makes Women Sick: Gender and the Political Economy of Health*. London: Macmillan.

Draper, J. (2014) 'Embodied practice: rediscovering the "heart" of nursing', *Journal of Advanced Nursing*, 70(10), 2235–2244.

Einstein, G. and Shildrick, M. (2009) 'The postconventional body: retheorising women's health', *Social Science & Medicine*, 69, 293–300.

Falcón, S. M. (2016) 'Transnational feminism as a paradigm for decolonizing the practice of research: identifying feminist principles and methodology criteria for US-based scholars', *Frontiers: A Journal of Women Studies*, 37(1), 174–194.

Fox, N. and Alldred, P. (2014) 'New materialist social inquiry: designs, methods and the research-assemblage', *International Journal of Social Research Methodology*. doi:10.1080/13645579.2014.921458

Fox, N. and Alldred, P. (2017) *Sociology and the New Materialism Theory, Research, Action*. London: SAGE.

Fraser, N. (2013) *Fortunes of Feminism: From State-Managed Capitalism to Neoliberal Crisis*. London: Verso.

Fraser, N. (2008) *Scales of Justice: Reimagining Political Space in a Globalising World*. Cambridge: Polity Press.

Freshwater, D. and Holloway, I. (2007) *Narrative Research in Nursing*. Oxford: Blackwell.

Fullagar, S. (2017) 'Post-qualitative inquiry and the new materialist turn: implications for sport, health and physical culture research', *Qualitative Research in Sport, Exercise and Health*, 9(2), 247–257.

Fullagar, S. and O'Brien, W. (2010) 'Rethinking women's experiences of depression and recovery as emplacement: spatiality, care and gender relations in rural Australia', *Journal of Rural Studies*, 58, 12–19.

Gibson, B., King, G., Teachman, G., Mistry, B. and Hamdani, Y. (2016) 'Assembling activity/setting participation with disabled young people', *Sociology of Health & Illness*. doi:10.1111/1467-9566.12496

Gill, N., Singleton, V. and Waterton, C. (2017) 'Care and policy practices', *Keele University: Sociological Review Monographs*, 65.

Gill, R. and Orgad, S. (2015) 'The confidence cult(ure)', *Australian Feminist Studies*, 30 (86),324–344.

Hankivsky, O. (ed.) (2011) *Health Inequities in Canada: Intersectional Frameworks and Practices*. Vancouver, BC: UBC Press.

Hankivsky, O. (2012) 'Women's health, men's health, and gender and health: implications of intersectionality', *Social Science & Medicine*, 74, 1712–1720.

Haraway, D. (1988) 'Situated knowledges and the science question in feminism and the privilege of partial perspective', *Feminist Studies*, 14(3), 575–599.

Haraway, D. (2008) *When Species Meet*. Minneapolis: University of Minnesota Press.

Harding, S. (ed.) (2004) *The Feminist Standpoint Theory Reader: Intellectual and Political Controversies*. London: Routledge.

Hekman, S. (1990) *Gender and Knowledge: Elements of a Postmodern Feminism*. Cambridge: Polity.

Hesse-Biber, S. N. (ed.) (2012) *The Handbook of Feminist Research: Theory and Praxis*. London: SAGE.

Hesse-Biber, S. N. (2014) *Feminist Research Practice: A Primer* (2nd ed.). London: SAGE.

Hesse-Biber, S. N. and Leavy, P. (2008) *Handbook of Emergent Methods*. London: SAGE.

Hill Collins, P. (2000) *Black Feminist Thought: Knowledge, consciousness, and the Politics of Empowerment* (2nd ed.). London: Routledge.

hooks, b. (1982) *Ain't I a Woman: Black Women and Feminism*. London: Pluto Press.

Hui, A., Schatzki, T. R. and Shove, E. (eds.) (2017) *The Nexus of Practices: Connections, Constellations, Practitioners*. London: Routledge.

Jackson, A. Y. and Mazzei, L. A. (2012) *Thinking with Theory in Qualitative Research: Viewing Data Across Multiple Perspectives*. London: Routledge.

Jaggar, G. (2015) 'The new materialism and sexual difference', *Signs: Journal of Women in Culture and Society*, 40(2), 321–341.

Janes, J. (2016) 'Democratic encounters? Epistemic privilege, power, and community-based participatory action research', *Action Research*, 14(1), 72–87. doi:10.1177/1476750315579129

Lather, P. (1991) *Getting Smart: Feminist Research and Pedagogy With/In the Postmodern.* London:Routledge.

Lather, P. (2015) 'The Work and Thought and the Politics of Research (Post) Qualitative Research'. In Denzin, N. and Giardina, M. (eds.), *Qualitative Inquiry and the Politics of Research.* London: Routledge, pp. 97–118.

Lather, P. (2016) 'Top Ten+ List: (Re)Thinking Ontology in (Post)Qualitative Research', *Cultural Studies ↔ Critical Methodologies*, 16(2), 125–131.

Lather, P. and St Pierre, E. A. (2013) 'Post-qualitative research', *International Journal of Qualitative Studies in Education*, 26(6), 629–633.

Latour, B. (2007) *Reassembling the Social: An Introduction to Actor-Network-Theory.* Oxford: Oxford University Press.

Leavy, P. (2017) *Research Design: Quantitative, Qualitative, Mixed Methods, Arts-Based and Community-Based Participatory Research Approaches.* London: The Guildford Press.

Letherby, G. (2003) *Feminist Research in Theory and Practice.* Buckingham: Open University Press.

Lupton, D. (2019) 'Toward a more-than-human analysis of digital health: inspirations from feminist new materialism', *Qualitative Health Research.* doi:10.1177/1049732319833368

Lupton, D. and Schmied, V. (2012) 'Splitting bodies/selves: women's concepts of embodiment at the moment of birth', *Sociology of Health & Illness*, 35(6), 1–14.

Kuhlmann, E. and Annandale, E. (2012) *The Palgrave Handbook of Gender and Healthcare* (2nd ed.). Basingstoke: Palgrave Macmillan.

Maller, J. C. (2015) 'Understanding health through social practices: performance and materiality in everyday life', *Sociology of Health & Illness*, 37(1), 52–66.

Maller, C. and Stengers, Y. (eds.) (2019) *Social Practices and Dynamic Non-humans: Nature, Materials and Technologies.* Maidenhead: Palgrave Macmillan.

Mertens, D. M. (2007) 'Transformative paradigm: mixed methods and social justice', *Journal of Mixed Methods*, 1(3), 212–225.

Mohanty, T. C. (1988) 'Under Western eyes: feminist scholarship and colonial discourses', *Feminist Review*, 30, 61–88.

Mol, A. (2008) *The Logic of Care: Health and the Problem of Choice.* London: Routledge.

Palmer, V. J., Weavell, W., Callander, R., Piper, D., Richard, L., Maher, L., Boyd, H., Herrman, H., Furler, J., Gunn, J., Iedema, R. and Robert, G. (2018) 'The participatory zeitgeist: an explanatory theoretical model of change in an era of coproduction and codesign in healthcare improvement', *Medical Humanities.* doi:10.1136/medhum-2017-011398

Phipps, A. (2014) *The Politics of the Body: Gender in a Neoliberal and Neoconservative Age.* Cambridge: Polity.

Puig de la Bellacasa, M. (2017) *Matters of Care: Speculative Ethics in More Than Human Worlds.* Minneapolis: University of Minnesota Press.

Ramazanoglu, C. and Holland, J. (2002) *Feminist Methodology: Challenges and Choices.* London: SAGE.

Reinharz, S. (1992) *Feminist Methods in Research.* Oxford: Oxford University Press.

Roberts, H. (1992) *Women's Health Matters.* London: Routledge.

Ryan-Flood, R. and Gill, R. (eds.) (2010) *Secrecy and Silence in the Research Process: Feminist Reflections.* London: Routledge.

Smith, L. T. (2012) *Decolonising Methodologies: Research and Indigenous People.* London: Zed Books.

Springer, K. W., Hankivsky, O. and Bates, L. M. (2012) 'Gender, health: relational, intersectional and biosocial approaches: Introduction', *Social Science & Medicine*, 74, 1662–1666.

St Pierre, E. A. (2015) 'Practices for the "new" in the new empiricism, the new materialisms, and post qualitative inquiry'. In Denzin, N. & Giardina, M. (eds.), *Qualitative Inquiry and the Politics of Research*. London: Routledge, pp. 75–96.

Tamboukou, M. (2008) 'A Foucauldian approach to narratives'. In Andrews, M., Squires, C. & Tamboukou, M. (eds.), *Doing Narrative Research*. London: SAGE.

Taylor, C. and Hughes, C. (2016) *Posthuman Research Practices in Education*. London: Palgrave Macmillan.

Tong, R. (2013) *Feminist Theories: A More Comprehensive Introduction* (4th ed.). Boulder, CO: Westview Press.

Walby, S. (2011) *The Future of Feminism*. Cambridge: Polity.

Warin, M. (2014) 'Material feminism, obesity science and the limits of discursive critique', *Body & Society*, 21(4), 48–76.

Wang, C. C. (1999) 'Photovoice: a participatory action research strategy applied to women's health', *Journal of Women's Health*, 8(2), 185–192.

Woodiwiss, J., Smith, K. and Lockwood, K. (2017) *Feminist Narrative Research: Opportunities and Challenges*. London: Palgrave Macmillan, Springer.

11

THE REFLEXIVE AUTOETHNOGRAPHER

Alec Grant

Introduction

There are a couple of things I'd like to say to you at the beginning of this chapter, to help you engage with my take on reflexivity when utilizing autoethnography, and in making these introductory points I am indebted to the work of Wanda Pillow (2003). Firstly, if you intend to develop your levels of autoethnographic reflexivity, you will need to keep in mind the following question: how does who I am, who I have been, who I think I am, and how I feel affect my autoethnographic inquiry? Secondly, at a more general level, never forget that the purpose of reflexivity is to address issues of power in the production of your autoethnographic work. This is done by critically and self-consciously making visible in it the practices of its production, at implicit or explicit levels.

I want to start this chapter by helping you shift out of your comfort zone. I will introduce reflexivity as a way of challenging your possibly habitual, un-scrutinized ways of thinking about your life and autoethnographic research, given that there should be no distinction between either of these areas. I will then go on to unpack the reflexivity concept in terms of what I regard as its most important component parts: critical (or ethico-) reflexivity, strong reflexivity and intersectional reflexivity. Following this, I'll take issue with the philosophical and conceptual bases of reflexivity in its context of use in humanistic forms of qualitative inquiry. This will be a good platform for me to proceed to argue that incorporating posthumanist diffraction into our reflexive sensibilities makes for more productive, creative, engaging and interesting autoethnographic work. This happens as we shift our epistemological goals from producing secure knowledge according to pre-determined onto-epistemological categories to striving for new, and potentially more troubling, forms of knowing and producing knowledge. In bringing the

The reflexive autoethnographer   197

chapter to a close, I will cover what for me are the key issues inhibiting the worthwhile practice of autoethnographic reflexivity-diffraction.

Get out of your rational mind

BOX 11.1 THE REFLEXIVITY KOAN

The last thing a fish notices is the water it's swimming in.
What do you think about what you think about?
What do you think about the way you think?
What do you feel about these things?
What do you think about these questions?
What do you feel about these questions?
The knowledge you produce is
produced by the knowledge that's
producing you.
And what do you think about that?
And how does it make you feel?
Reflexivity is not solipsism.
Neither is it self-awareness.
Self awareness seduces humanists. However,
self awareness makes zero onto-epistemological sense and
a pre-occupation with such naval gazing keeps you at sea;keeps your eyes off the
bigger deal;
stops you from experiencing yourself in the world
and the world in you.
Hold your head up.
Look out, look back, but don't look down.
Humanists assume the truth of
The lone, Romantic, Enlightenment Self,
ontologically prior to
its inscription within
social structure, relationship, dialogue.
Humanists don't get out enough,
or think enough,
or read enough, or, perhaps,
feel enough.
Instead, they float around on the sea
of their own impossibilities.
Reflexivity is postmodern, poststructural, performed, courageous.
Reflexivity is cultural interpretation.
Reflexivity is cultural engagement.

198 Alec Grant

> Reflexivity gets you out of the box, out of the cave, onto dry land and into life.
> And what do you think about that?
> And how does it make you feel?
>
> *(Grant, 2013, pp. 38–39)*

A koan is a narrative or poetic device used in Zen Buddhist practice. Its purpose is to help practitioners drop their habitual over-reliance on reason by engaging them in paradoxes. I wrote the Reflexivity Koan to use in my postgraduate qualitative inquiry teaching in the face of what I perceived to be a 'dumbing down' agenda – at least in healthcare research education (Grant, 2013). I wanted to help students grasp the implications of the experiential as well as the rational dimensions of reflexivity in qualitative inquiry. In so doing, I also wanted to trouble their taken-for-granted ways of thinking and feeling, and their tacit and automatic acceptance of commonplace but insufficiently challenged ways of construing the world of healthcare research.

Moreover, I wanted to go beyond the conventional understanding of reflexivity as a 'turning back' in a researcher's writing to explore her or his reciprocal impact on the research field and participants. I hoped that the koan might lead at least some students to appreciate and *perform* reflexivity in broader, deeper and more methodologically coherent ways, through encouraging them to address the levels of *paradigm, philosophical and theoretical governing principles, methodology, methods, narrative content* and *relational ethics* in their work. How well *you* perform reflexivity in your research will depend on your levels of critical self-consciousness across all of these areas. Below, I hopefully demonstrate such comprehensive reflexive engagement in the context of, mostly but not exclusively, my own writing.

At this point however, I want to help you better understand the Reflexivity Koan. It begins by inviting readers to consider an aphorism voiced by the communication theorist and philosopher, Marshall McLuhan. Just as a fish takes for granted the water it lives in, so people tend not to step back from and question the content of their thoughts, their styles of thinking and corresponding emotions. How often do *you* do this? I believe that such questioning is fundamental to autoethnographic reflexivity.

The koan proceeds to address reflexivity at the level of *philosophical and theoretical governing principles*, in the onto-epistemological assertion that no researcher construes reality or produces knowledge in a vacuum. You, me and everyone else engaged in qualitative inquiry are more or less constrained by taken-for-granted assumptions and structures of power. These work to shape and delimit our scholarship, research, writing practices, and institutional, professional and methodological allegiances, some or all of which have insufficiently challenged 'sacred cow' status. Unless we do reflexivity by questioning, challenging, and, when necessary, working against these assumptions and power structures, we are in danger of reducing autoethnographic inquiry to a one-

The reflexive autoethnographer   199

dimensional technical activity that fails to live up to its methodological brief of cultural interrogation.

The remainder of the koan is a call to *paradigm* reflexivity in its critique of humanism, or, more precisely, 'liberal-humanism'. In short, this term refers to assumptions of: the superiority of humans in the world over other animals and material phenomena; their cradle-to-grave developmental coherence; their ability to look accurately at a world which is always, as it were, outside of them; and their default tendency to reflect on what they see and hear, in order to make rational choices in the interests of their own betterment. I suggest instead in the koan that what we habitually assume about coherent, atomized selves is a fiction, and that who we are at any point in space in time depends – in post-human and new materialist terms – on the socio-material assemblages within which we are entangled (Grant, 2016a, 2018a, 2018b). These contexts are always power-imbued and, as I argued in the previous chapter, constitute 'culture' (Grant, 2018a, 2018b; Grant et al., 2013). I will proceed to unpack these points more in the context of a definitive look at autoethnographic reflexivity.

Autoethnographic reflexivity

You will recall from Chapter Nine that the need for researchers to attend more to human rather than colonizing stories, and to let go of the stance of omniscient but absent researcher, emerged as a consequence of the crisis of representation. Being autoethnographically reflexive thus requires you to shift from objective and rational – sometimes called 'malestream' – research sensibilities to those associated with feminist inquiry. The demand on you is to reveal rather than conceal your emotions, other embodied and relational lived-experiences, and self-conscious autoethnographic practices, within your research (Holman Jones et al., 2013).

Critical reflexivity (or ethico-reflexivity)

This means that relational ethical considerations are *always* going to be implicated in performing reflexivity. As Carolyn Ellis (2007) argues, *critical reflexivity* is inseparable from the process of writing autoethnography. In using this term, she is referring to *the constant internal struggle, or dialogue, we have with ourselves about how we represent ourselves and others in our research.*

Ellis reminds us that autoethnography entails a 'flip-flopping' movement between experiencing and examining a vulnerable self, and revealing the broader social context of that experience. Accepting the general ethical principle that social relationships should be protected as much as is reasonable, Ellis cautions that the choices we make about what and who to include in our writing can have the effect of improving or damaging those relationships. This does not imply simple binary, either-or, decisions aimed at sanitising our work to the extent that it is *always* social damage-free. Your work will inevitably offend some readers (Grant, 2018a). However, it does mean that if you intend to craft autoethnography, you can never be absolved from the discomfort of what I prefer to describe as 'ethico–reflexive' self-dialogues and choices.

To illustrate this, let's revisit a quote from my own work from the previous chapter; see Box 11.2.

BOX 11.2 DRINKING TO RELAX

His shoes crunch the shingle on the short path as he slowly lumbers towards his council house. At sixty, looking seventy-five, he carries the sadness of four decades of bad marriage and chronic unfulfillment. Stooped, obese, arterio-sclerotic, hungover, laboured breathing in time with short pinch-toe gait, he trudges reluctantly to the front door. Anticipatory defensive anger builds and quickly turns his face from default red to puce. Three short steps to go as, sweating, he prepares for the onslaught. Key in the lock now. Turn slowly. Open door quietly. There she is. Dash meets Peg. Peg meets Dash. As usual. Only this time Peg is not ranting vitriol at full volume. Only this time Peg is dead dead not dead drunk. Purple face meets purple face. Two yards from the front door, feet off the ground, her body swings obscenely in this final Fuck You goodbye moment.

(Grant, 2018b, pp. 33–34)

Of all my writing to date, the ethico-reflexive challenges for me in crafting the 'Drinking to Relax…' paper were enormous. How did I deal with those?

BOX 11.3 ETHICAL CONCERNS

Crafting this piece has helped me move my own story on, but I am left with ongoing concerns around how I've represented those no longer around to respond to my portrayal of them. I'm aware that by writing about my mother, father and brother, I've fallen foul of this ethical issue in order to stamp my own story with rhetorical authority. Ironically given my earlier criticisms of how I experienced their treatment of me, I've trapped them in my own narrative.

That said, sense making after suicide inevitably means that the stories of those who take their own lives, and others implicated in this, are narratively re-colonised by those left behind … Since dialogue was never a feature of my life with my mother, brother or father when they were alive, who they

The reflexive autoethnographer **201**

> were for me is how I experienced and remember them. They were and are
> for me what they did.
>
> *(Grant, 2018b, pp. 39–40)*

In line with my argument in the previous chapter about the functions and purposes of autoethnography, and with a constant awareness of the demands of reflexivity at the levels of *methodology, methods* and *narrative content*, I felt compelled to write and publish this autoethnography to better understand my early life and, at least to some degree, liberate myself from it. In terms of ethico–reflexivity at a theoretical level, I also wanted to further explore '…narrative entrapment in imposed biographies' (Grant, 2018b, p. 33), in keeping with my already published autoethnographic work in this area (Grant & Leigh-Phippard, 2014; Grant, Leigh-Phippard, & Short, 2015). Moreover, in terms of reflexivity at the levels of *paradigm, theory* and *philosophy*, I felt the need to provide analytical and sociological depth to my story by analysing it using New Materialist principles (see Box 11.4).

BOX 11.4 NEW MATERIALIST ANALYSIS

At an abstract conceptual level, New Materialism does not regard good or bad 'health' – psychological, physical, or relational – as embodied attributes of individuals. Instead health assemblages are processes connecting bodies to their social and broader material environments. This is achieved through flows of affect, which simultaneously enable and limit the capacities of bodies to act, think and desire. In Drinking to Relax, affect flows can be seen to gain relative stability through their transgenerational consolidation. They are also place-, time- and class-based, gendered, learned and over-rehearsed to the extent that they seemed 'natural' to my mother, father, brother, myself and other characters in the story.

. . . my mother was constrained to do her drinking behind closed doors, living as she did within arguably an even narrower range of relational and network possibilities. Ways out of this for her were extremely limited – a situation that clearly worsened throughout the story, making her decision to take her own life understandable.

Moreover, her death, and the described emotional difficulties that she and I, and my brother and father in less acknowledged ways, had in life, are intelligible in the context of intergenerational trauma as affect flow. From a New Materialist perspective, emotionality is simultaneously embodied, performed, and relationally, materially, and transgenerationally distributed. Houses, towns, family and individual reputations, and reduced possibilities of becoming-other, are component parts of negative emotional assemblages. My mother had a lifetime history of personal misery, was unhappy in her marriage, and – certainly in the social groups she lived among, and the generation she came from – divorce was never a possibility in mid-20th century small town Highland life.

(Grant, 2018b, pp. 42–43)

However, I violated the cultural ethical taboo about writing critically about the dead, and did this in graphic, visceral and profane ways. That said, in terms of *ethico-reflexivity towards narrative content,* I believe that cultural taboos against auto/biographically negative obituaries (Grant, 2017a, 2018b) need to be robustly challenged. I hoped that by doing so, my work would add to the qualitative knowledge base of trauma-inducing and oppressive family relationships and offer new ways of thinking about such relationships. This points us in the direction of 'strong reflexivity'.

Strong reflexivity

Anderson and Glass-Coffin (2013) argue that strong reflexivity should occur in the context of the researcher's in-depth and heightened awareness of their connection to the research situation and their impact on it. These authors describe strong reflexivity as a form of researcher introspection informed by an ethical need to constantly strive towards a better understanding of self and others. They argue that this is achieved through an explicit examination of one's perceptions, actions and reciprocal dialogue with others.

Anderson and Glass-Coffin mention the common strategy of achieving strong reflexivity by describing and reflecting on one's self across different points in time and cultural contexts. The autoethnographic story in *Drinking to relax . . .* contains vignettes portraying me in my social and material home life circumstances at various points in time from the mid-1960s to the late-1970s. I found writing the story in this way extremely valuable in achieving and portraying an in-depth 'understanding of the fragmented, and temporally and contextually shifting nature of selves and relationships' (Anderson & Glass-Coffin, 2013, p. 73; see Box 11.5).

BOX 11.5 DEMONSTRATING STRONG REFLEXIVITY

In so many ways, I'm grateful that my mother functioned for me as a negative role model. Although double-edged and experienced sometimes as a tyranny more than a virtue, I have spent much of my adult years writing against intra- and inter-personal violence, often simply experienced and viewed by many people as just the way the world is. So, in my academic work I try to expose forms of 'narrative entrapment' whenever and wherever I can. I use this term to refer to the phenomenon of people being held captive in the stories imposed on them by others and by themselves. This can happen in families, where individuals are caught up in forced biographies to the extent that they come to believe and self-identify with oppressive stories, told about them by one or both parents, and sometimes by siblings and people in the wider community. . . . Narrative entrapment can also happen at institutional, organizational and public levels, when, for example in the name of mental health treatment, many people are given diagnostic labels that more or less guarantee futures characterized by discrimination, stigma and being treated as less than fully human . . .

In recent years this has led to my growing interest in story telling as social and human science, and, hopefully, utilizing such stories in the service of social justice. Quite simply, writing about significant aspects of our lives helps us re-story ourselves, in terms of finding who we are and the direction in which we are moving our lives forward. Such writing has helped myself and others become more aware of and work towards our preferred identities . . . and to critique the narrative entrapment characteristic of stagnant, un-scrutinized lives. . . . The therapeutic function of re-storying narrative identity . . . and the developing international importance of autoethnographic voice, story transmission, and personal transformational writing . . . helps us make better and different sense of painful and distressing life experiences. As an ethical act of self-compassion, re-storying helps reclaim biographies, purge burdens, and determine what kinds of lives could and should be lived. We are all made expert by our own experiences, and writing our lives arguably enables us to become increasingly sophisticated in this regard.

(Grant, 2018b, p. 39)

Intersectional reflexivity

The quote in Box 11.5 directly points, as I argued in the previous chapter, to the need for the reflexive autoethnographer to develop their 'sociological imagination' (Wright Mills, 1959), to identify the 'systems that shape, constrict, disrupt . . . (and) . . . inform both the story and the storyteller' (Pathak, 2010, p. 8). However, a note of caution is perhaps warranted here: if you have aspirations to reflexively explore a political standpoint from an imagined monocultural identity, you will soon come to realise that you actually occupy several cultures simultaneously, and that these don't always happily cohere together. Reflexive autoethnographic writing therefore needs to be informed by *intersectional* theoretical considerations.

Intersectional theory (see, e.g. Crenshaw, 1989, 1991; Crenshaw & Harris, 2009) refers the ways in which our writing is always inscribed within multiple and conflated, historical, cultural contextual and discursive circumstances (Grant 2018a). To put this in hopefully a more straightforward way, irrespective of

204 Alec Grant

what time period we find ourselves in, we are *always* performing life according to lots of shifting, often mutually contradictory and conflicting, cultural influences that give rise to our experience of ourselves. In this regard, the work of Renata Ferdinand (2018) constitutes a masterful exemplar of intersectional reflexivity, and also displays the coming together of *theoretical governing principles, methodology, methods, narrative content* and *relational ethics* in a powerful and dramatic way (see Box 11.6).

BOX 11.6 DEMONSTRATING INTERSECTIONAL REFLEXIVITY

I recently presented an autoethnographic essay on the life of Renisha McBride at an academic conference. I nervously stood at the podium and began with the following proclamation:

I died today. It wasn't because of . . . illness that somehow managed to ravage my 19-year-old body. It wasn't due to an unfortunate circumstance of . . . falling . . . while building a pyramid with my cheerleading team . . . surprisingly, I died from a single gunshot wound to the face from a 12-gauge shotgun.

I looked at the audience members and saw the . . . look of surprise on their faces, but continued,

Never mind that I banged on the door of a stranger. . . . It shouldn't matter that this was in the suburbs. . . . I only sought help.

I could hear the rustling of uncomfortableness as audience members nervously shifted from left to right in their seats . . .

But help did not come. I was not afforded the care given to other accident victims. No ambulance rushed me to the hospital. . . . Instead, I lay dying on the front porch of . . . Theodore Wafer's house. In the early morning dawn, the silence and stillness of the neighbourhood was interrupted by the . . . bang of a shotgun.

I would go on to tell the audience her story . . . comparing it to the plight of black women and the problems that arise when we ignore the intersection of being black and female. I wanted the audience . . . to know her story . . . her death was virtually unnoticed. compared to other deaths at the time . . .

Initially the audience was quiet, so I anticipated little to no questions. But . . . one audience member . . . seemed to speak for them all. . . . She plainly asked, "Who are you to tell her story. . . . Did you even know her? Do you know her family? You tell a really good story, but your story would be deeper if you sought . . . to learn more details about her life and her death. . . . You're a storyteller, and in keeping with West African culture, you are responsible for remembering . . . keeping traditions . . . preserving history . . . you need to see her family. . . . Go further. I'm assuming that everyone had the same suggestions because they all nodded in agreement.

> . . . "That's good advice. I'll see what I can do." . . . Secretly, I boiled inside. .
> . . I felt diminished and defeated. Her thoughts stayed with me: Who did I think
> I was? I know what my intent was – I wanted McBride's story to be used to
> highlight the struggle of black women . . . noting their invisibility . . .
>
> *(Ferdinand, 2018, pp. 149–151)*

From reflexivity to diffraction

Although indispensable for good autoethnographic work, you should be aware that when used as a *humanist* methodological tool, reflexivity signals sensitivity to the portrayal of normative and reliable socio-cultural identities and categories of experience. Pillow (2003) reminds us that a driving assumption of humanist-informed reflexivity is of subjects and researchers who are singular, knowable and improvable through research. The nature, variation and nuances of these identities and categories, always already either known or anticipated, have been the staple of qualitative inquiry over the decades. In reflexive humanist writing, people are given close-scrutiny, centre-stage presence, with nature, the material and non-human animals forming a kind of narrative backdrop (Grant, 2016a).

Now, If I and the people I write about are knowable, then clearly what is needed are better methods of reflexivity to *know better*. But this may simply reinstitute and reproduce exactly the hegemonic structures that need to be worked against by autoethnographic researchers operating within a social justice agenda. In contrast, an emphasis on diffraction moves us in a different, *posthumanist,* direction (Grant, 2016a, 2018b). This facilitates the emergence of the novel rather than the familiar, in work where the usual boundaries between humans, non-humans, and the material, organic and inorganic collapse.

Understanding the people, other animals and things represented as multiple, unknowable and constantly shifting, changes the purposes and practices of autoethnographic inquiry, and thus reflexivity. Moreover, writing from the perspective of human and non-human others does not necessarily involve finding things in common with them. In lots of respects I am never confident that I know myself very well, let alone other people. Erin Manning (in Massumi, 2015, p. 145), arguing from a broadly posthumanist standpoint, asserts that 'The biggest mistake we make is to pretend that we can categorize and compartmentalize events according to pre-established criteria.' I take her words to mean that the use of humanistic onto-epistemological categories in the service of 'reflexivity' has significant political consequences. It seems to me that the use of pre-determined, normative categories of subjectivity and other aspects of the world often signals reflexive habit and tired repetition rather than the creative emergence of the new, novel, unfamiliar, transgressive and challenging.

206 Alec Grant

Given this, I would urge you *not* regard or dismiss diffraction simply as a device to shock. In my own work, I aspire to write diffractively while also attempting to maintain fidelity with the sentiments of reflexivity. I do this by striving to both find new ways of *performing* narrative autoethnography and creating takes on the world that I did not have prior to writing, which emerge through it. Being surprised by my own writing, and developing and changing myself and the world as a result of it, is an autoethnographic gift for me, and I hope you have similar experiences in your own work.

I should stress at this point that in the reflexive-diffractive autoethnographic quest to improve our worlds, multiple perspective witness accounts of these worlds at particular points in time-space are better narrative resources than futile attempts to write *the truth*, irrespective of qualified, humanist epistemological claims for situated knowing. In both postmodern versions of reflexivity and posthumanist diffraction, the aim is not to achieve certainty – quite the opposite. Reflexivity-diffraction is always about self-conscious, situated, partial, and uncertain but valuable knowing in an uncertain world. As Pillow (2003, p. 180) argues, '…using reflexivity to write toward the familiar works against the critical impetus of reflexivity and thus masks continued reliance upon traditional notions of validity, truth, and essence in qualitative work.'

Lisa Mazzei (2014) celebrates the significance and importance of diffraction in the need to trouble the longstanding and habitual practices of conventional qualitative inquiry described above. She argues that the basis of these practices in a general strategy of mechanistic coding and reducing data to themes robs storied life of its entangled complexities, richness and surprises. In response to this state of affairs, and in line with the seminal work of Karen Barad (2007), Mazzei (2014, p. 742) argues for diffraction as a highly productive methodological strategy of 'reading insights through one another'. This phrase refers to thinking about qualitative data with social, human and other scientific theoretical concepts in multi-layered ways, where these theoretical concepts are 'plugged into' data (Jackson & Mazzei, 2012). This allows for a better, richer, more entangled and complex portrayal of life through emergent and unfolding, shifting, unpredictable and unfamiliar, thoughts, meanings and juxtapositions. If you engage with it, diffractive writing will help you productively transgress normative epistemological assumptions and practices through producing knowledge differently and producing different knowledge (Klevan et al., in press).

I hopefully demonstrate such diffraction-in-autoethnographic action in Box 11.7. In a quote from work which interweaves autoethnographic data with posthuman philosophy and theory, I also make deliberate strategic use of the Japanese prose-poetry form – 'haibun' – and allude to the work of the English poet Philip Larkin. I do so to add to the dramatic content of my paper and, hopefully, also demonstrate my commitment to self-conscious *narrative reflexivity*.

BOX 11.7 DEMONSTRATING DIFFRACTION AND NARRATIVE REFLEXIVITY

. . . boyfriends come and go in the same repeated pattern. Each relationship begins in harmless and mundane ways. For many weeks, they meet in neutral territory: in restaurants, on walks, normal stuff.

Then comes the time when she will invite him home, at which point she gets increasingly needy, as well as taking on all his interests. If it goes far enough, if he's lucky, he makes it upstairs. Getting upstairs reasonably quickly will help him see more clearly. He then starts to cool off, wanting distance. In response to this, she will become more and more desperate and clingy. He will try to end things gently and amicably without hurting her, but will not be allowed to succeed in this.

'Such a rotten shame.
All her boyfriends are bastards.
Treating her badly.'
This is how we've lived.
This is our family home,
welcoming you in.

Washing sheets by hand.
Like we've always had to.
No place for machines.

Upstairs, my bedroom.
My accumulated life.
My so precious world.

The house
Suspicious ramparts:
all back stories scrutinised,
of those who enter,
No life allowed that's
unpleasant and unruly,
soiling certainties.

Nobody welcomed
who doesn't fit the decor,
clashing with its scheme.
The house judges him,
moral foundations shaking,
finding him guilty.

> She dies of cancer in 2016, after the longest, seven year, spell of not speaking to him. As usual, refusing to have any truck with death, even though for her it was three years in the making, it transpires that she never made a will. So in weeks after her burial, he helps his wife clear out the family house, as part of the bigger task of the disposal of her assets.
>
> He has never felt welcomed by it. Being simultaneously dead and alive, the house has pores. Out of these seep decay. Through these, he is sucked as he walks reluctant through the front door. Immediately absorbed into its foetid, sweet-smelling stickiness, a nasty cloying in his throat registers his assimilation and causes him to gag a little. He smells decay and damp – the kind of smell that belongs more in abandoned slums than a recently vacated mid-terrace house.
>
> He holds himself together and looks around. Piles of stuff lie everywhere, with very important things, like doctors' letters, in amongst the trivial. Receipts for items bought and long forgotten and random notes to no-one in particular, written long ago. Detritus in neat heaps deepening, coastal shelf-like, down the years.
>
> He clocks the piles of seashells and rocks – in jars, in pots, on shelves. Jammed between photo albums, much more than there used to be. Much more than he imagined there could me. Old clothes on hangers, over every door and bannister. Upstairs is worse, her bedroom worst of all.
>
>
> Flotsam and jetsam,
> tried on, not worn, piled up, and
> forever waiting
>
> Afterwards, back home,
> he strips his clothes, moist and soiled.
> Hot shower, bad sleep . . .
>
> *(Grant 2017a, pp. 62–63)*

I anticipate that you will have read my words in the quote in Box 11.7, and in this chapter more generally, in situated and shifting ways, and this will obtain if you go back to the chapter at different points in the future (Grant, 2018a). Does my reflexive self-consciousness evoke reader self-consciousness in you? When I speak to you directly in the second person, do my textual interruptions evoke textual interruptions in you; as you unavoidably re-story my narrative? Do I make you feel uncomfortable?

Conclusion: inhibitors of autoethnographic reflexivity-diffraction

In bringing this chapter to a close, I want to say to you that I strongly agree with Pillow (2003) when she argues that the practice of reflexivity should be uncomfortable. What does she mean by this? There are several possible answers to this question that you might want to consider in the context of your own work. In Pillow's terms, reflexivities of discomfort serve the general purpose of knowing the world better, while always, as discussed above, situating such knowing as tenuous and uncertain. Knowing is interrogated and provisional, and multiple answers and perspectives are provided or implicitly invited of audiences by authors. So, auto-ethnographic reflexivity-diffraction needs to be used in a kind of contradictory way, to continue to challenge the representations of the world we make while at the same time acknowledging the political need to always represent and find meaning.

Extending on Pillow's work, I believe that 'reflexivities of discomfort' is also a good descriptor of an autoethnographer's attempt to self-consciously undermine conventional representational practices by troubling cultural sacred cows. In this regard, I have in this and my previous chapter deliberately used my own work to show the ways in which it goes against the grain of cultural normativity, including the tacit convention of always storying the dead in eulogistic terms.

Further, it follows that discomfort reflexivity work needs to challenge conventional narrative representational practices in terms of the overall form and vocabulary content of texts. In regard to the former, the editorial practices of some healthcare journals have the effect of 'shoehorning' autoethnographic work into conformity with positivist article structuring guidelines (Grant, 2016b). The obvious danger of this is that much of the creativity of such work gets lost or camouflaged in the process.[1]

Turning to vocabulary content, and with an eye to my previous chapter in this volume, it is ironic that the uncritical acceptance and reproduction of master stories such as the one of 'mental illness' is displayed by many qualitative researchers in healthcare. This might be regarded as a form of 'narrative habitus', or habitual use of certain words and phrases. It's not unusual to see work by mental health writers making rhetorical appeal to authority and neutrality while uncritically using the language, vocabulary and tropes of the master narrative of mainstream, orthodox psychiatry. This points up a contradiction between these writers' explicit or implicit claims to paradigm and narrative reflexivity and their clinging on to anachronist, scientifically discredited and power-imbued ways of describing human psychological distress (Grant, 2015; Grant & Gadsby, 2018; Smith & Grant, 2016). If you sign up to discomfort reflexivity, you can never be too careful over your choice of words.

This points to a potentially more disturbing issue: the power that healthcare institutions, organizations and professions either possess or have been granted by autoethnographers, to set limits on how much we can critique our jobs, organisations, professions and institutional allegiances in our work. At this point, I'll remind you of an assertion I made earlier in this chapter: 'No researcher

---

1   To illustrate this point, you may want to read my co-written work employing 'messy text' representational practices (Short et al., 2007), and consider what would be gained and lost by structuring this text in a conventional way.

construes reality or produces knowledge in a vacuum. You, me and everyone else engaged in qualitative inquiry are more or less constrained by taken-for-granted assumptions and structures of power. These work to shape and delimit our scholarship, research, writing practices, and institutional, professional and methodological allegiances'. If you are, for example, being funded by your organization to conduct your research, how free or otherwise do you feel you can be to critique this organization in your work, and, at a deeper level, critique the assumptions that govern its practices? And how comfortable are you about directly revealing yourself in such critiques?

BOX 11.8 TOILETS ARE THE PROPER PLACE FOR OUTPUTS

It's mid-July, 2016 and I'm presenting my work at the University of Brighton's annual Teaching and Learning Conference. Its title this year is 'Nurturing Co-Construction,' and the 30 or so delegates at my session are mostly University of Brighton academics, some of whom I know very well as they work in my school.

I start my presentation in a light-hearted way by disclosing that I'm in my last 10 months before retirement and old-age pension, so it's a privilege to be able to reflect on what I think has been one of the most gratifying areas of my 20-plus years as an academic in higher education. I disclose that I've recently been passed over for a professorial appointment, which might not have been the case had I been more of a 'big bucks' research grant enthusiast. They laugh when I say that the kind of 'grant attraction' that interests me the most is the one where the students I work with are attracted to researching and writing with Alec Grant, who is likewise attracted to doing this with them...

In the hour or so before my conference slot, I rehearsed what I hoped would be a hubris-busting statement: 'I'm very proud about the "impact" our work has made, in what for me is the best sense of the term. When I first heard my publications described as "outputs" by a professor in my school whose role was to increase our Research Excellence Framework (REF) scores, I had the immediate thought that toilets are the proper place for outputs! This raises a few giggles among delegates when I say it, and I wait for the laughter to die down before mustering the necessary gravitas to go on to tell them 'I'm talking about impact in the sense of our writing being helpful for people and the development of useful knowledge.'

(Grant, 2017b, pp. 45–46)

As the quote in Box 11.8 illustrates, I personally don't have a problem with the demonstration of institutional, professional and organizational discomfort reflexivity. This is also evidenced by my recent critical autoethnographic work based on my lived-experiences as a mental health educator (Grant, 2013, 2016c, in press; Grant and Radcliffe, 2015), writing mentor (Grant, 2017b) and autoethnography mentor (Klevan et al., in press).

Does this make me very different from you? I will never know the answer to that question. What do you think? I am by disposition a risk-taker in my autoethnographic writing, and I'm relatively unconcerned about the fallout on my career and its development now that I'm an independent scholar with no career to develop. At the risk of sounding pompous and stereotypically autoethnographic, I like to think of myself as having always been a critical thinker, driven less by a desire for social approval than by the need to write truth to power. So, perhaps it's appropriate for me to end this chapter by answering the question I posed for you at its beginning: how does who I am, who I have been, who I think I am, and how I feel affect my autoethnographic work? My answer is *in every way*!

References

Anderson, L. and Glass-Coffin, B. 2013. I learn by going: Autoethnographic modes of inquiry. In: Holman Jones, S., Adams, T.E. and Ellis, C. (eds.), *Handbook of Autoethnography*. Walnut Creek, CA: Left Coast Press, 57–83.

Barad, K. 2007. *Meeting the Universe Halfway: Quantum Physics and the Entanglement of Matter and Meaning*. Durham, NC: Duke University Press.

CrenshawK. 1989. Demarginalising the intersection of race and sex: A black feminist critique of antidiscrimination doctrine, feminist theory and anti-racist politics. *University of Chicago Legal Forum*, 1989, Article 8: 139–167.

Crenshaw, K. 1991. Mapping the margins: Intersectionality, identity politics, and violence against women of color. *Stanford Review*, 43(6): 1241–1299.

Crenshaw, K. and Harris, L. 2009. A primer on intersectionality. *African American Policy Forum*: http://aapf.org/wp-content/uploads/2013/01/59819079-Intersectionality-Primer. pdf

Ellis, C. 2007. Telling secrets, revealing lives: Relational ethics in research with intimate others. *Qualitative Inquiry*, 13: 3–29.

Ferdinand, R. 2018. Getting it out there: (Un)comfortable truths about voice, authorial intent, and audience response in autoethnography. In: Turner, L., Short, N.P., Grant, A. and Adams, T.E. (eds.), *International Perspectives on Autoethnographic Research and Practice*. London and New York: Routledge, 148–156.

Grant, A. 2013. Writing, teaching and survival in mental health: A discordant quintet for one. In: Short, N., Turner, L. and Grant, A. (eds.), *Contemporary British Autoethnography*. Rotterdam, Boston and Taipei: Sense Publishers, 33–48.

Grant, A. 2015. Demedicalizing misery: Welcoming the human paradigm in mental health nurse education. *Nurse Education Today*, 35: e50–e53.

Grant, A. 2016a. Storying the world: A posthumanist critique of phenomenological-humanist representational practices in mental health nurse qualitative inquiry. *Nursing Philosophy*, 17: 290–297.

Grant, A. 2016b. Researching outside the box: Welcoming innovative qualitative inquiry to nurse education today. *Nurse Education Today*, 45: 55–56.

GrantA. 2016c. Living my narrative: Storying dishonesty and deception in mental health nursing. *Nursing Philosophy*, 17: 194–201.

Grant, A. 2017a. Writing the dead in two parts. In: Sparkes, A. (ed.), *Auto/Biography Yearbook 2016*. Nottingham: Russell Press, 55–72. Available at www.researchgate.net/profile/Alec_Grant/contributions

Grant, A. 2017b. Toilets are the proper place for 'outputs'! A tale of knowledge production and publishing with students in higher education. In: Hayler, M. and Moriarty, J. (eds.), *Self-Narrative and Pedagogy: Stories of Experience within Teaching and Learning*. Rotterdam: Sense Publishers, 45–57.

Grant, A. 2018a. Voice, ethics, and the best of autoethnographic intentions (or writers, readers, and the spaces in-between). In: Turner, L., Short, N.P., Grant, A. and Adams, T. E., eds. *International Perspectives on Autoethnographic Research and Practice*. London and New York: Routledge, 107–122.

Grant, A. 2018b. Drinking to relax: An autoethnography of a highland family viewed through a new materialist lens. In: Sparkes, A. (ed.), *Auto/Biography Yearbook 2017*. Nottingham: Russell Press. Available at www.researchgate.net/profile/Alec_Grant/contributions

Grant, A. In press. Moving around the hyphens: A critical meta-autoethnographic performance. In: Williams, S. (ed.), *Critical Mental Health Nursing*. Monmouth: PCCS Books.

Grant, A. and Leigh-Phippard, H. 2014. Troubling the normative mental health recovery project: The silent resistance of a disappearing doctor. In: Zeeman, L., Aranda, K. and Grant, A. (eds.), *Queering Health: Critical Challenges to Normative Health and Healthcare*. Ross-on-Wye: PCCS Books, 100–115.

Grant, A. and Radcliffe, M. 2015. Resisting technical rationality in mental health nurse higher education: A duoethnography. *The Qualitative Report (TQR)*, 20(6), Article 6: 815–825. Available at www.nova.edu/ssss/QR/QR20/6/grant6.pdf

Grant, A. and Gadsby, J. 2018. The power threat meaning framework and international mental health nurse education: A welcome revolution in human rights. *Nurse Education Today*, 68: 1–3.

Grant, A., Short, N.P. and Turner, L. 2013. Introduction: Storying life and lives. In: Short, N.P., Turner, L. and Grant, A. (eds.), *Contemporary British Autoethnography*. Rotterdam: Sense Publishers, 1–18.

Grant, A., Leigh-Phippard, H. and Short, N.P. 2015. Re-storying narrative identity: a dialogical study of mental health recovery and survival. *Journal of Psychiatric and Mental Health Nursing*, 22: 278–286.

Holman Jones, S., Adams, T. and Ellis, C. 2013. Introduction: Coming to know autoethnography as more than a method. In: Holman Jones, S., Adams, T.E. and Ellis, C. (eds.), *Handbook of Autoethnography*. Walnut Creek, CA: Left Coast Press, 17–48.

Jackson, A.Y. and Mazzei, L.A. 2012. *Thinking with Theory in Qualitative Research: Viewing Data across Multiple Perspectives*. London and New York: Routledge.

Klevan, T., Grant, A. and Karlsson, B. In press. Writing to resist; writing to survive: Conversational autoethnography, mentoring, and the new public management academy. In: Moriarty, J. (ed.), *Writing to Resist, Writing to Know: Autoethnographies from Higher Education*. London and New York: Routledge.

Mazzei, L.A. 2014. Beyond an easy sense: A diffractive analysis. *Qualitative Inquiry*, 20(6): 742–746.

Massumi, B. 2015. *Politics of Affect*. Malden, MA: Polity Press.

Pathak, A.A. 2010. Opening my voice, claiming my space: Theorizing the possibilities of postcolonial approaches to autoethnography. *Journal of Research Practice*, 6(1). Available at http://jrp.icaap.org/index.php/jrp/article/view/231/191

Pillow, W.S. 2003. Confession, catharsis, or cure? Rethinking the uses of reflexivity as methodological power in qualitative research. *Qualitative Studies in Education*, 16(2): 175–196.

Short, N., Grant, A. and Clarke, L. 2007. Living in the borderlands: Writing in the margins: an autoethnographic tale. *Journal of Psychiatric and Mental Health Nursing*, 14: 771–782.

Smith, S. and GrantA. 2016. The corporate construction of psychosis and the rise of the psychosocial paradigm: Emerging implications for mental health nurse education. *Nurse Education Today*, 39: 22–25. Available at http://authors.elsevier.com/a/1SXhbxHa58Ccw

Wright Mills, C. (1959/2000). *The Sociological Imagination: Fortieth Anniversary Edition*. New York: Oxford University Press.

INDEX

agency 7, 12, 13, 85, 144, 165, 179, 183, 190–191
autoethnography 159; analysis 160; definitions 160–162; dissemination 172; evaluating 171–172; forms of 160; and narrative writing 160–162; limits and critiques of 172–173; politics and philosophy of 162–171
awareness 135–136

Barad, K. 183, 185, 189–190, 206
Bennett, J. 183, 187
bias 29; *see* ideological pragmatism
binary, binary thinking, binaries 13, 180, 183, 199
Braidotti, R. 13, 183
Buddhism 129, 134–135

case study methodology 41; analysis 45, 48–50; history 41–42; types of case study design 42–43; case protocol 44–46; critiques 50; examples 42, 43, 46
Charmaz, K. 73–75, 77–78, 82, 95, 101, 104
concepts of social change 7, 14, 186, 188, 189, 191
consciousness 120, 128–129; philosophical and psychological theories of 129–132; *see* neurophenomenology
constructionism, constructionist, constructivism 8, 12, 75
Corbin, J. 73, 77, 95, 98
critical histories of qualitative and qualitative health research 6–10

critical qualitative research 2, 3–9
critique of qualitative research 9–10; autoethnography 165; case study 50; ethnography 144; feminism 179–180; feminist research 180–181; grounded theory 72–74, 88, 98–100; humanism 165, 179, 199; phenomenology 113–114; participatory narrative 182

data methods 53–70; data analysis 65–66, 68; grounded theory 72–73
decolonising research 8–9, 111
Denzin. N., Y. Lincoln. 165–166
dimensional analysis 96–101
discourse analysis 37–38
dissemination of qualitative health research 32–34; of autoethnographies 172–173
documents as data 66–68

Ellis, C. 199–200
embodiment 116, 119, 188, 190; *see* phenomenology
epistemology 10, 91; as interpretative 42; as modern and postmodern 165; as ontoepistemology 184; as posthuman 14; as relativist 74, 91; in ethnography 150; in grounded theory 95; in phenomenology 116
ethics 12, 13, 16, 55, 58, 79, 198, 204
ethnography 142–144; history of 146–149; *see* focused ethnography
European enlightenment 11–12

Experience, lived experience 132–135; *see* phenomenology

feminism 7, 9, 10, 20, 95, 177–178; and philosophies, politics and practices 178–181; and feminist theories 177–179; and feminist research practices 180–183; and postcolonial, post structural feminism 178–179; and material feminist theories and research 183– 186; examples of 187– 190; limits of 190–191
fieldwork in healthcare research 53; access and conduct in 63–66
focused ethnography 152 –153, 154–155
focus groups 61–62

gender and gendered relations 178, 179, 201; in feminist research 180, 186
Giorgi, A. 111–112, 117, 127
Glaser, B. 72–75, 76–78, 81, 82, 83, 95
grounded theory 71–90, 91–109; grounded theory terminology 94; and analysis 76–78, 84; and constant comparison method 76; and dimensional analysis 96–101; and history of 72–75; and literature review 84–86; memo writing 81–82, 103–104; reflexivity 82; theoretical sampling, sensitivity and saturation 76, 80; writing a grounded theory 86–88

Haraway, D. 14, 183
Heidegger, M. 114, 126–127, 137
histories of qualitative research 6–10
Holman-Jones, S. 169–170, 171
humanism 12–13, 179, 187, 190, 191
Husserl, E. 110, 111–114, 126, 128, 131, 134, 137, 147

idealism 129–130, 137
ideological pragmatism 26–29
indigenous research 7, 8–9, 179, 185, 191
interpretative 12, 73, 78, 181; interpretative phenomenology 114; interpretative phenomenological analysis 30, 127
intersectionality 179, 180; intersectional reflexivity 203–205
interviews 54–61; virtual interviewing 58–61

Lupton, D. 189–190

material feminism 20, 177, 180; and analysis 185–190, 201; theories and philosophies 183, 185–187; limits of 190–191

materialism 126, 132, 177, 185, 191; as monism 129–130
methodology 10, 54, 55, 63, 146, 149, 155, 181; diffractive methodology 184; methodology and case study 41– 44, 50; methodology and ethnography 146, 149, 150; methodology and grounded theory 71–72, 81, 92–94, 95; methodology and phenomenology 116, 127; methodology and researcher position 26–28, methodology and reflexivity 198, 201, 204
methods 3–6; in ethnography 154, 155, in feminism 181, 188; *see* data methods
Mol, A. 189

narrative research 181–182; narrative turn, narrative healing, narrative recovery 168–169
National Health Service 142, NHS, primary care and public and patient engagement and involvement 142–144
neoliberalism in healthcare 1, 9, 15–16, 164–165, 177–179, 189
neurophenomenology 120–121
new materialism, new materialisms 20, 183

objectivity 7, 12, 53, 73, 178
observational methods 62–63
ontoepistemology 184, 185

participatory research 182–183
phenomenology 110–124, 125–141; phenomenology as research; analysis 114–116 bracketing 114, 119, 126–128; bridling 113; contemporary directions in *see* neurophenomenology; descriptive phenomenology 111, 113–114; hermeneutic /interpretative phenomenology 116, 126
philosophical positions 90–92, 93; philosophy as practices 150
philosophy 8, 10–15; and consciousness 129; and continental 118; and Eastern 136; and phenomenology 112–116, 126; and posthumanism 165, 208
politics 15–16
postcolonial 7, 10, 11, 178–179; in participatory research 182–183
posthumanism 12–14, 16, 19–20, 165, 183; in more–than–human–world research 185–186; in autoethnographic reflexivity 199; as diffraction 205–207 and critical

216 Index

poststructuralism, poststructural 7–9, 11, 20, 179, 180, and poststructural feminism 183, 190; and narrative research 182–183, 186, 187

power 5, 7–8, 15–16, 209–211; cultural power 165; explanatory power 98; feminist research 179–183, 188, 196, 198; in poststructural research 15, 165; research position 91

practices of qualitative research 16, 53–70

practice theory 14, 144, 155, 183; practice theories 144 –146; practice theories and analysis 145, 151

qualitative data analysis 74, 76, 79–82, 85, 92, 100

qualitative methods 3–6, 15, 17, 27, 28, 29, 31, 43, 48, 53–54, 67–68, 93–94, 110, 119, 150; *see* interviews; interviewing

qualitative research and philosophies 10–15; *see* qualitative methods; data methods

queer theory, research and activism 7, 8, 9, 10, 11, 178, 183; *see* critical theory, critical qualitative research 3–6

realism 180; realist 16–18, 31, 33, 42, 74, 95, 135, 155, 165, 186–187; agential realism 190; and ontology 91; naïve realism 167; 170

reflexivity 34–35; in autoethnography 196–213; grounded theory; feminist and material feminist research; intersectional reflexivity 203–204; phenomenological research; reflexivity and diffraction 205–208; strong reflexivity 202–203

Schatzman, L. 71, 78, 96

sensitive subjects 60–61

Shove, E., M. Pantzar, M. Watson 144

social constructionism, social constructivism; *see* constructionism

socio-material theories *see* practice theories

Stake, R.E. 43–44

Strauss, A. 65, 71–72, 73, 77, 101

subject, subjecthood, 12–14, 55, 120, 126; in research 62, 74, 186, 205; subject and object 129–130; 185–186

subjectivity 12, 13–15, 102, 126, 131, 134–138, 173, 181, 182, 188, 190–191; healthy subjectivities 188; intersubjectivity 116, 153; normative subjectivity 205; transcendental subjectivity 128

thematic analysis 30–32, 36; and critical discourse analysis 37

triangulation 46–48

voice 7–8, 67–68, 75; authorial voice 82; in feminist research 194–95; presenting voices 113; reclaiming voice 170; representing voices 147, 180–182; suppressing voice 173

Wenger, E. 145

Wenger, E., B. Traynor 155

Yin, R.K. 43–44, 45, 48